MASTERING MINDFULNESS

A self-discovery journal
And behavior change program
To conquer weight loss
And create a life of balance

be INSPIRED | *be* EMPOWERED | *be* MINDFUL

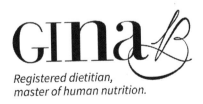

Registered dietitian,
master of human nutrition.

Copyright © 2017 Gina Worful Nutrition, Inc. All rights reserved.

This book, or any portion thereof, may not be reproduced or used in any manner whatsoever without the express written permission of the publisher, except for the use of brief quotations in a book review.

Contributors:
Zack Prager, MAPP, Founder of Ransomly
Heather Foat, Founder of Liv4Yoga

The nutritional information in this book is not intended to be a substitute for professional medical or psychological advice, diagnosis, or treatment. Always seek the advice of your physician, or another qualified health provider, with any questions you may have regarding a medical condition. Never disregard professional medical advice or delay seeking it because of something you have read in this book.

Printed in the United States of America

Thank you to all of the amazing people who have supported me during my journey toward mastering mindfulness. I am beyond grateful for my clients who have welcomed me into their lives, allowing me to understand them and to help me become a better dietitian. Thank you to all of you who have given me your unconditional support. I am ecstatic to finally have an outlet to share my passion with you.

Who is Gina B?

Gina Worful, MS, RD is recognized as Gina B – helping you *be* INSPIRED and *be* EMPOWERED to be your best self yet. She is a registered dietitian with a master's degree in human nutrition from one of the top dietetics programs in the country at Eastern Michigan University. Her notable research review on "Ending the Destructive Eating Cycle" and a multitude of client success stories have led to the development of this *Mastering Mindfulness* book. Gina speaks across the country with presentations for Morgan Stanley, Stardock Corporation, and the world-renowned health spa, Cal-a-Vie Spa Havens. Gina has helped hundreds of people overcome their diet struggles and reconnect to their bodies through mastering the principles of mindfulness.

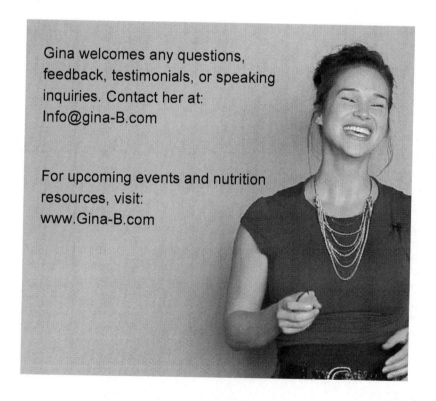

Gina welcomes any questions, feedback, testimonials, or speaking inquiries. Contact her at:
Info@gina-B.com

For upcoming events and nutrition resources, visit:
www.Gina-B.com

Preface

I decided to explore the concepts of mindfulness after seeing so many people consistently failing with their structured meal plans. I saw them filled with frustration and self-doubt. When I started speaking and teaching workshops on mindfulness, I saw faces light up throughout the room. People were having their own "aha" moments from thought-provoking questions that no one had ever asked them to consider. They each had unique struggles and experiences, but they realized that their common denominator was the deeper self-imposed limitation they had created, not a lack of willpower that they were made to believe that they had. Seeing their "light bulb" moments inspired me to continue to help people further their self-realization to accomplish the impossible.

Mastering Mindfulness will address how your eating, environment, and thinking have an impact on your overall health and happiness. You will have the opportunity to non-judgmentally explore why, what, how, when, and with whom you eat. In addition, we will dive into strategies related to your eating habits, cravings, and how to properly fuel your body using science-backed nutrition information. Throughout this journey, I hope you experience your own amazing "aha" moments and share them with your friends, family, and even me. From the bottom of my heart, I hope you are inspired, empowered, and more mindful after reading this book.

Contents

Introduction	1
What is Mindful Mastery?	5
But Does Mindfulness Work?	6
Why the Health Industry is Failing Us	9
The Weight Loss Struggle	14
Tapping Into Your Why-Power	21
Part 1: Exploring the Past	25
Is All This Exploring Actually Important?	27
Mindful Eating: What are your food memories?	39
Mindful Living: Where have you struggled?	46
Mindful Self-Talk: What was your self-perception?	54
The Power of Positivity	61
Part 2: Observing the Present	63
Mindful Eating	65
What Did You Learn?	82
Social Situations	86
Mindful Living: What can you control?	87
Mindful Self-Talk: How do you talk to yourself?	93
Part 3: Planning for the Future	97
Mindful Eating	99
Mindful Living	132
Mindful Self-Talk	147
FAQ	156
Mindfulness Mastery Plan	159
Bibliography	167

Introduction

Master your mind and you can master anything. It is estimated that adults are faced with an average of 35,000 decisions in one day. If you allow your emotions, other people, and your own thoughts create self-imposed limitations you will feel helpless in making the best decisions for yourself. Do you...

- Struggle with sticking to a healthy diet or having control over your food?
- Feel stress from work, life, and your relationships?
- Talk down to yourself about the way you look or the choices you make?
- Set goals but continuously sabotage them?

If you answered yes to any of those questions, this program is ideal for you. *Mastering Mindfulness* will help you gain control over your thoughts and become empowered to change your habits that shape your future. This isn't a typical book that you read passively, learn from, and use to possibly make a few changes once you're finished. This book will give you a self-discovery experience that has the potential to change your life entirely. This step-by-step program will guide you to:

1. Explore pieces of your past
2. Observe your current habits
3. Create a customized plan to conquer your biggest struggles in the future.

You will be writing in this book, so make it YOUR book. Get comfortable putting your pen to paper. Start by taking the Mindfulness Self-Assessment on the next page to evaluate your current level of mindfulness.

Mindfulness Assessment	Rarely (3)	Sometimes (2)	Always (1)
I enjoy the present moment		2	
I don't worry about the future or the past			1
I feel in control over my food choices	3		
I eat until just content, not stuffed or still hungry		2	
I can leave food on my plate if I feel content		2	
I eat slowly without distractions and put my fork down in between bites	3		
I say positive and encouraging things to myself when I make mistakes or don't stick to my diet		2	
I can observe my feelings without getting lost in them		2	
I pause and think before reacting to situations			1
I allow myself to sit with or experience difficult feelings			1
I make the time and space for things that make me happy			1
I take quiet time to explore my thoughts and feelings without TV, music, a computer, or other distractions			1
Totals:	6	10	5

Total score: _____ 21

Score of 26 – 36: High need for mindfulness training
Score of 15 – 25: Moderate need for mindfulness training
Score of 12-14: Low need for mindfulness training

If you scored in the 26-36 range, then mindfulness might be very new to you. Don't be discouraged if changing these habits seems like a lot to take on. I will be guiding you every step of the way toward reconnecting with your body and becoming a Mindful Master!

If you scored in the 15-25 range, then you might already be using some of the principles of mindfulness, with some areas needing a little focus or practice.

If you scored in the 12-14 range, you are probably doing a good job of listening to your body's needs and practicing mindfulness daily. This program will be beneficial to further explore your habits and continue sharpening your self-awareness and mindfulness practice.

Having the patience to complete this program will give you the opportunity to non-judgmentally explore and gain a deeper understanding of your habits. At every moment our thoughts, physical body, and experiences change. When people say that you were acting out of character or "not like yourself," – well, that authentic self doesn't really exist. With new information entering our minds at every second, we can't be expected to think and act the same as we once did. So know that self-study should be an ongoing practice, not an endpoint to be reached.

There is truly no relationship more important to understand than the one you have with yourself. Once you become aware of your own patterns, habits, and thoughts, you can stop your mind from being a self-sabotaging enemy, and turn it into a powerful tool in reshaping your future. You can understand how and why you respond to certain situations to have full control in changing the outcome. If you feel that the relationship with yourself has fallen to the wayside, or maybe never really existed, know that it is never too late to start. Just like any bad or neglected relationship, it takes time to listen, understand, and trust again. And that's where *Mastering Mindfulness* comes in.

==This book is like an adult coloring book: If you don't put in the time to color in the pages of the journal with your observations and experiences, your results will be just as blank.== However, if you explore your habits and note your observations, you will see progress. You will learn to listen to what your body needs so you ==intuitively== know when and how much to eat. You will be empowered to eat healthy foods and have indulgences in control, without feelings of guilt. Instead of letting fear or anger guide your actions, you will have full control over your emotions, enabling you to free yourself from stress and create better relationships with those around you.

==By shifting your mindset, you will break down self-imposed limitations to take control of your future.== You will be able to transform your thoughts to fully embody a positive and self-loving person. Together, we will uncover the struggles you have battled and release old habits to make space for change. By committing to this program, you will learn more about yourself and be able to break through barriers more successfully than with any food plan alone. This will all be done by practicing mindfulness. There are three components to *mastering mindfulness*: *mindful eating, mindful living,* and *mindful self-talk.*

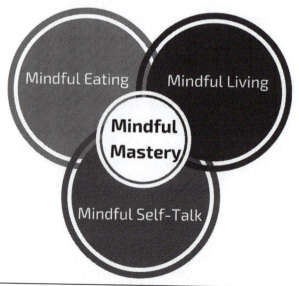

What is Mindful Mastery?

Mindfulness is being present in the moment by having awareness of your mental and emotional state and thoughts that will direct your purposeful actions.

Mindful eating is aiming to eat slowly in order to enjoy fully the sight, smell, texture, and taste of food while remaining aware of internal levels of hunger, fullness, and satisfaction (also known as satiety). By practicing mindful eating, you'll regain control over intense cravings, manage your weight easily, and end bingeing or frequent overeating.

Mindful living is being fully aware and staying in the present moment, not letting the past or future create unnecessary anxiety and worries. Living mindfully will help you let go of what you can't control in order to help reduce stress, so that you can see important problems that need to be addressed. Being present in the moment can improve your communication and relationships with others, and give you the freedom to live with intention and purpose. *THIS IS VERY IMPORTANT*

Mindful self-talk is being aware of the thoughts and attitude we have toward ourselves. Positive and loving self-talk will improve your confidence and put a stop to self-sabotaging behaviors.

Mindful is the opposite of mindless.

But Does Mindfulness Work?

Mindfulness techniques have been practiced more than two thousand years to create an experiential awareness of the present moment. Countless studies support the benefits of mindfulness practice including improved mental focus and attention, positive immune and cardiovascular health, weight management, lower levels of depression and anxiety, prevention of mood disorders, emotional regulation, improved sleep, and decreased pain. The following table lists only a handful of the many studies that support the benefits of practicing mindfulness.

Benefit	Study	Results
Focus and Memory	*Mindfulness training improves working memory capacity and GRE performance while reducing mind wandering.*	A two-week mindfulness training showed improvements in Graduate Record Examinations (GRE) scores and working memory capacity. The training also reduced the occurrence of distracting thoughts, which led to improved cognitive performance.
Improving Sleep Disturbances	*The relationship among mindfulness, rumination, and stress-related sleep disturbance*	A correlational analysis of 153 college students found that mindfulness interventions that develop presence, non-judgment, and acceptance may help improve stress-related sleep disturbance.
Immune System Health	*Lymphocyte recovery after breast cancer treatment and mindfulness-based stress reduction therapy.*	Women receiving Mindfulness Based Stress Reduction Therapy had significantly higher recovery of T cells 12 weeks after cancer treatment versus those with usual care.

Cardiovascular Health	*The effects of Mindfulness-Based Stress Reduction on cardiac patients' blood pressure, perceived stress, and anger: a single-blind randomized controlled trial.*	Cardiac patients receiving Mindfulness Based Stress Reduction Therapy had significant reductions in systolic blood pressure, perceived stress, and anger than the control group.
Enhanced Awareness of Hunger and Satiety Cues	*Body and mind: mindfulness helps consumers to compensate for prior food intake by enhancing the responsiveness to physiological cues.*	Mindful eating interventions resulted in participants' abilities to naturally adjust to caloric needs based on previous intake of meals compared to poor adjustments made from less mindful eaters.
Portion Control	*Does mindfulness matter? Everyday mindfulness, mindful eating and self-reported serving size of energy dense foods among a sample of South Australian adults.*	Participants who reported daily mindfulness practices at higher levels of mindful eating and reported smaller serving size estimates of food.
Reducing and Managing Depression and Anxiety	*Journal of Clinical Psychology*	Reduction in depression relapse from 78 percent to 36 percent when Mindfulness-Based Cognitive Therapy was added to traditional treatment.
Emotional Regulation and Confidence	*A conscious control over life and my emotions: Mindfulness practice and healthy young people. A qualitative study.*	Data showed that mindfulness practice created greater calm, balance, and control. It also created a mindset of greater confidence and competence while lessening the risk of future distress.

Beyond the data and studies, I have been helping clients for years resolve their food struggles, feel empowered, and regain their confidence through *mastering mindfulness*. These are only a few of the many who have used the principles of mindfulness to create a life they can thrive in:

"I feel less stress and more in control than I ever have. I haven't been on a scale since July, but I have a doctor's appointment tomorrow and hope the scale is nice. My tight jeans fit great last week." – Sharon

"With small changes, I went from starving all of the time, to being happy and satisfied with my meals and snacks. I'm eating foods I love, as well as eating foods I'd never tried before. We all know food isn't always about being hungry. Now I notice my triggers and am able to cope with stress-eating before I end up bingeing. Chocolate is just an occasional treat and not the daily focus." – Susan

"For the first time in longer than I can remember, I'm not writing down (i.e., stressing out over) every single thing that I eat. I've taken a completely new approach to my lifestyle, and I can honestly say I've never felt happier about the choices I'm making. I am still learning, and I have a long way to go to reach my goals, but I know I will succeed." – Chris

"Over the course of about a year, my eating habits have changed significantly for the better, without ever feeling 'forced' to change or having to 'drop what I loved eating.' I've also gained a very healthy desire for exercise. I am doing more physical activities just for fun, and I have just integrated them into my lifestyle." – Roger

Why the Health Industry is Failing Us

While having a structured eating plan can be a useful tool to guide our food choices, most diet programs fail to acknowledge that we aren't so simple. Mindfulness gives us the ability to understand our behaviors, making it the foundation for living healthfully. Whether the goal is to create a healthy life transformation, lose weight, or regain control over food, solely relying on a meal plan will almost always ultimately result in failure.

When starting a new diet, many people end up quitting not too long after and, as a result, become consumed with frustration and guilt for not sticking to their plan. If you're blaming yourself too, know that it's not entirely your fault. Changing your eating habits is far more complex than just having enough willpower. Your own environment, the diet plan that you're trusting, and mega food companies could be mentally and physically sabotaging you until you fail. A serious pitfall of diet programs is their lack of tools to effectively re-pattern eating behaviors.

Creating new habits must become an integrated part of the lifestyle in order to stay sustainable. Otherwise, established habits will perpetuate and automatic behaviors will continue. We live in a fast-paced world that disconnects our mind and body. Your body might be screaming for what it needs but it easily gets drowned out if you have to jump out of bed at 6 A.M., get ready for the day, take care of kids or pets, rush off to work, do a never-ending list of errands, clean, cook dinner, pay bills, do the recommended 45 minutes of exercise, catch up with friends, and keep your family happy.

Over time we forget to a) tune in to our body's needs and hunger cues, b) be aware of internal stress and live in the present moment, and c) listen to our self-talk. With life so busy, we ignore what our body is telling us and turn to quick-fix diet programs when healthy eating has been neglected. We become reliant on diets with strict rules and use destructive self-talk as our "motivation." Most people take this route because it seems much easier than taking the time to tune inward and understand our habitual, emotional, and environmental triggers that sabotage goals. Unfortunately, this approach rarely ever works long-term.

New meal plans with a different angle and promising transformational results pop up just about every week; but if it were as easy as just following "the plan" why would we fail? If they did work, the need for new ones would go away and the struggle to be healthy would no longer be a focus in our society. Sticking to a healthy diet seems to be the most popular challenge that people have in common. Most people have, at some point, tried a diet or two – or ten – only to find themselves failing over and over again.

How many times have we heard the "I'll just start over again on Monday?" Or how about "After this cookie, I'll never eat another one again!" Sound familiar? Creating change is much more complex than just having the willpower to not eat unhealthy foods. Having a meal plan with food rules doesn't dig deep enough into why we sabotage our goals. In order to truly conquer your struggles, it's important to understand where they come from in the first place.

Think about the caveman days, when food had to be hunted or gathered. Cavemen never knew if they were going to be able to find food, make it through the weather extremes, or have to fight off a wild animal. This situation was both challenging and stressful, but the stress gave them the innate drive to seek food for survival.

Fast-forward to today. We still have those same instincts for seeking out food in times of stress. We might not be fighting off lions, but we do have families, finances, work or school, our health, deadlines, relationships... the list goes on. So our natural instincts tell us to eat for comfort and survival.

To make matters worse, food is incredibly easy to get these

days. Most people can just drive to the store or a fast food restaurant, open up the kitchen cupboards for a snack, or pick up the phone for a delivery to get just about any food quickly. On top of all that, we are up against food companies that spend billions of dollars in advertising and creating foods that are so incredibly delicious that it becomes nearly impossible to stop eating. These food companies try to formulate their recipes to create a "bliss point" – the perfect combination of sugar, fats, salt, and flavorings that creates a euphoric eating experience. Maybe that's why Lay's has coined the slogan "Betcha can't eat just one" since 1963. Food companies commonly create an addictively flavored food and pair it with an ad campaign or slogan that tugs at our heartstrings. Here are a few trademarks that you may recognize:

"Help yourself to happiness." – Golden Corral
"The best taste for the best times."– Stouffer's
"There's a lot of joy in Chips Ahoy!" – Kraft Foods
"Life's better the Milky Way." – Mars
"Unleash the Joy." – Mars
"Crack into an unforgettable Dove chocolate experience." – Mars
"When you need a moment, chew it over with Twix." – Mars
"You deserve it!" – Mars
"Have a little fun anytime." – Mars
"Colorful chocolate fun!" – Mars
"Great flavor! More fun!" – Frito-Lay
"Good vibes start with great flavor." – Frito-Lay
"Packed full of smiles." – Frito-Lay
"Make break time happy time." – Frito-Lay
"Lay's. Brighten your day." – Frito-Lay
"Keep smiling." – Frito-Lay
"Happiness in every bite." – Frito-Lay
"Happiness in every crunch." – Frito-Lay
"The taste that brings us together." – Frito-Lay
"See the flavor, taste the rush." – Frito-Lay

"Lay's get your smile on!" – Frito-Lay
"Come hungry, leave happy." – IHOP
"Love at first bite." – The Food Network
"Sip on some inspiration." – Coca-Cola
"Open happiness." – Coca-Cola
"Taste the feeling." – Coca-Cola
"Get happy." – Coca-Cola
"Taste the love." – Coca-Cola
"Consuming this product may cause joy." – Coca-Cola
"Unwrap a new you." – Hershey Chocolate
"Indulge in chocolate bliss." – Hershey Chocolate
"Put a smile on your face." – Hershey Chocolate
"Making memories for a lifetime." – Hershey Chocolate
"Every day deserves a kiss." – Hershey Chocolate

This list could continue for pages. Companies push the message that you deserve to eat their treats to escape stress and feel happy. ==Now, isn't it clear to see how easily we can get emotionally attached to food?==

Between instinct, easy accessibility, and the strategic influence of mega corporations, it can be very challenging to eat a healthy, balanced diet without our environment sabotaging us. We are also hounded by the message that the only way to get healthy is through a strict diet. Here's what a typical "dieting cycle" looks like:

Day 1: "I am determined to do it this time! I am ready to start my journey to optimal health with this new diet plan!"

Day 2: "Okay, I'm starving… and kale sucks… but I'm still going to do it this time!"

Day 2.5: "Boy, I'd love a piece of chocolate right now… chocolate… chocolate… chocolate…. No, don't do it… maybe just a nibble… no, don't do it."

Day 3: "Chips! Candy! Chocolate! Pizza! Oh, how I've missed you so! NOM! NOM! NOM!"

Day 4: "Why did I do that? I feel so guilty... I'm never eating those foods again. Tomorrow, I'm starting over... back on my diet."

Are you a victim of this pattern? Don't worry, most people who diet are. Strict meal plans set you up for failure by expecting you to change your life completely, overnight. If you've spent your entire life creating your habits, you can't be expected to undo all of them and create new ones by the next day. It would be like asking you to go from couch potato to running a marathon all in the span of twenty-four hours. Running a marathon takes time and patience to build your endurance. Most people training might evaluate where they are starting from, set a goal for how far they need to go, and consistently add a mile each time they have conquered a new distance. Understand that I'm not suggesting you run a marathon, but to appreciate what it takes to make such a significant change.

Standard diet plans also don't consider your starting level of nutrition or cooking knowledge. Let's say you're excited to start this new "clean eating" or "quick fix" meal plan that gives you a list of foods you can and can't eat. On your "can list" you have quinoa and kale, which you may never have bought, cooked, or tasted, let alone know how to pronounce – but this is supposed to be your new way of eating by tomorrow. The "can't list" is full of all the foods you're familiar with and ones you know you'll miss. So what do you do? Inevitably, you'll go back to your comfortable old ways of eating. Changing the way you eat should be a fun journey of exploring the uncharted territory of new healthy foods and deciding which ones are a "go" and which ones are a "no."

The Weight Loss Struggle

While the sole purpose of *Mastering Mindfulness* is not weight loss, it does give you the ability to regain control over food and make better choices, which could result in healthy weight loss. If your goal is to lose weight, following a restrictive diet program physically works against your body, making long-term success incredibly challenging. When most people are highly motivated to lose weight, they drastically restrict their calories to quickly lose fat. What they don't realize is that their body is not only burning fat but it is also breaking down muscle for energy, because they aren't eating enough food. Your muscle is the main component of your metabolism because it burns the majority of the calories you eat while you're exercising, sleeping, sitting, or simply going about your day. The more muscle you have, the more calories your body will burn at rest. So, over time, drastically restricting how much food you eat can cause you to lose muscle and slow your metabolism.

Once you start losing weight, your body instinctively tries to bring you back to your original starting weight by influencing your appetite as a survival mechanism. Think of your body like a thermostat. It will release certain hormones to naturally increase or decrease your appetite to keep you as close to the same comfortable temperature (your body weight) as it possibly can. While many different hormones and mechanisms influence this physiological dance, ghrelin and leptin are two key players.

During weight maintenance, the role of ghrelin and leptin is to keep the body at a comfortable weight. Appropriate amounts of ghrelin are released before a meal to send hunger signals indicating that food is needed. Appropriate amounts of leptin are released toward the end of a meal to signal that enough food has been consumed to maintain energy balance in the body.

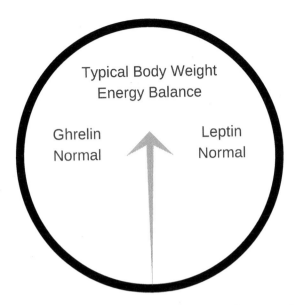

During calorie restriction, the body releases higher than normal amounts of the hormone ghrelin to intensify appetite and send the signal to eat more food. This encourages weight gain as a survival mechanism during times of weight loss. Once weight gain ensues, ghrelin can stay elevated for four weeks after the body returns to its "typical" weight.

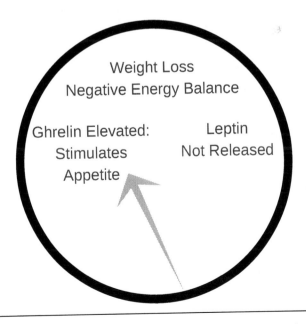

When you have had an ample supply of calories, your body releases the hormone leptin to soothe your appetite to signal you to stop eating.

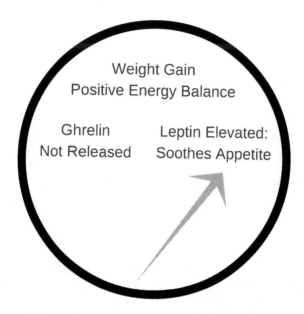

Unfortunately, the signal from leptin is much weaker than ghrelin so, it is easy to override the signal that you have had ample food and allow yourself to overeat anyway. The ghrelin signal has a strong effect on stimulating the drive to eat, making it very difficult to stick to a low calorie diet long-term. If you do eat extra calories and gain weight, this becomes your new normal weight (thermostat temperature) that your body tries to maintain.

This is why the typical outcome from strict dieting is that most people will end up bingeing on their favorite pre-diet foods a few days after they have started a new diet. The problem with cycles of restriction followed by overeating is that with a slower metabolism, the body can't keep up with the additional calories. You're much more likely to regain the weight you lost, and then some more! It's a vicious cycle that continually sets you up for failure, and the more you fail, the more you lose confidence and trust in your relationship with food. Food becomes the enemy.

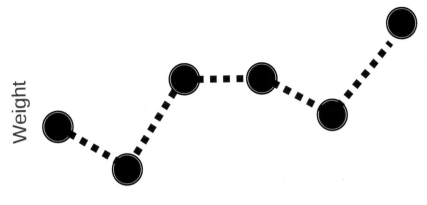

This pattern explains why many people have been diet experts for years but can't figure out why they weigh more than they ever have. If you keep following the pattern of starting and stopping restrictive diets, it is very likely that over time you will either gain weight or that maintaining your weight will only become more of a struggle. The key is to make gradual healthier changes that are not too overwhelming to integrate into your lifestyle and don't fire up your appetite-stimulating hormones. It's almost like tricking your body by gradually cutting back calories without alerting the hormone police!

We are all incredibly unique, so one basic quick-fix diet plan just cannot work for everyone. Let's say you're in a big group of people and each person takes off his or her left shoe and passes it to another person. If you try to put it on, it's not very likely to fit. That's exactly what fad diets are like! They give out the same "shoe size" to a variety of feet, and we wonder why they never work. Everyone has a different food preference, body type, metabolism, sensitivity to certain foods, medical conditions, level of motivation, experience with cooking, nutrition knowledge base, and goals. If you consider yourself a "foodie" who loves to cook, then your plan for eating healthier would be drastically different from someone who works long hours and needs grab-and-go meals.

Long-term success will be achieved when you take the time to discover foods that you will personally love *and* that will help you reach your goals. You'll then never want to quit that way of eating. The need for "willpower" goes away, and your new way of eating becomes a part of your life.

Truly changing your life for good requires self-exploration and a little patience along the way. Don't let all of this diet talk discourage you if you are eager to make changes or try a structured meal plan to get healthier. Taking this initiative is fantastic and I fully support you doing it, but only in the right way so you are successful. If you want to get healthier and don't know if you are making a lifestyle change or just doing a fad diet, ask yourself, "Could I eat this way forever?" If your answer is no, then you know it won't be sustainable. It's okay to use resources or meal plans for guidance on healthy eating, but you shouldn't feel like you are suffering and barely able to stick to it every day.

Successfully building new habits usually happens by taking on one to three goals at a time. When you focus on just a few goals, you can practice working it into your lifestyle without feeling overwhelming and wanting to quit. A goal might be to try a new healthy recipe, drink a certain amount of water, or cut out late-night snacking. Focusing on a few goals at a time creates more steady progress because the change is not so overwhelming that it causes the "quit and start over" cycle. Some spend one or two weeks practicing to incorporate the new goal into their life, until it naturally becomes a part of their daily routine, like brushing their teeth or showering. Then, they are ready to take on another goal or two.

When trying to make a change that has already been a lifelong habit, it could take months to years of practice. For example, if you have been a fast eater since childhood, it might take many months to practice slowing down. Those who take this slow and steady route are far more likely to be successful than those who try to suffer through a restrictive 1200-calorie meal plan. We will go into nutrition strategies in Part 3 to help guide you if you are trying to eat healthier during your journey toward *mastering mindfulness*.

This book will give you the step-by-step tools to regain control over food and finally conquer common eating struggles. Those who have a loss of control over food often repeatedly fail with diets because of uncontrollable cravings and feelings of hopelessness. Countless studies continue to show that overeating, stress, depression, and poor body image all feed into the repetitive cycle of restriction, followed by overeating that can feel impossible to get out of.

The Destructive Self-Sabotaging Cycle shows how our emotions, self-perception, and eating behaviors are interconnected. Dieting, in the form of calorie-restriction, is typically unsuccessful as a means of long-term weight control, resulting in continuous diet failures and feelings of depression. This depression triggers unhealthy eating behaviors, such as binging, night eating, and emotional eating, to ease the negative feelings associated with the failure. These eating behaviors create more self-doubt and stress. Feeling stressed releases cortisol, which physiologically spurs more cravings, triggering even more eating. This then creates negative self-talk about who you are, the choices you are making, and your inability to keep the promises you have made to yourself. The self-doubt makes you believe that you are not actually this "healthier and in control" person that you want to be, so your own mindset sabotages your goals and causes you to overeat. Do you see the cycle?

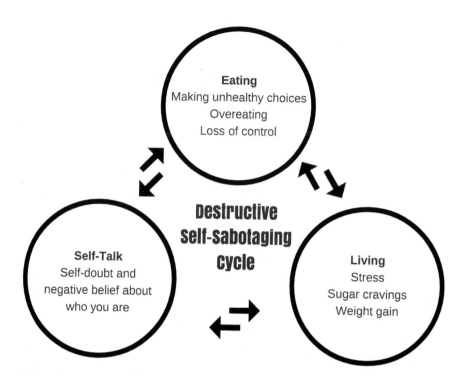

Healing each area of mindfulness – mindful eating, mindful living, and mindful self-talk – will allow you to end this destructive cycle. You can love what you eat without feeling stuffed and guilty, and embody a positive self-loving person. The key to long-term success lies in discovering your own personal weaknesses and gradually working toward building new habits that will lead to accomplishing your goals. You'll be able to conquer your own struggles and build new habits that you'll never want to give up.

Tapping Into Your Why-Power

Before you begin your journey, I want you to think of your "why." Why do you want to *master mindfulness* or create a change? It could be that you want to be healthier to keep yourself out of the hospital, feel less stressed, be more patient and happy when you're with your family, be more kind to yourself, or have the physical ability to climb a mountain or do the activities you love. A good friend of mine is considered a "snowmobile addict." Just about every weekend in the winter he's up north in Michigan to play in the powder. One day he said, "Who cares about being healthy? We're all just going to die anyway." He had a point but then I asked, "Can you snowmobile from a hospital bed?" I think he found his "why."

The purpose isn't to keep you alive forever, but to *expand* the time that you make your life the most fulfilling it can be and compress the time of illness. Having a greater purpose will drive forward your change. When many people come to see a dietitian, they usually are focused on the goal of losing weight. Unfortunately, the goal of weight loss isn't ingrained deep enough into our hearts to create a profound motivation that long-term change requires. Having the commitment to change old habits can come from two different scenarios:

1. Something entirely rocks your world. Maybe you were diagnosed with pre-diabetes or an illness, you saw an old photo of a younger and healthier you, or a life moment happens that impacts you so intensely that you make the commitment to change and never look back. Ninety-nine percent of people will never have a significant enough experience to create the permanent mental shift. If you're part of the majority, you would follow scenario 2…

2. You make the commitment to change but in a more patient, exploratory way. Most people don't want this method because they don't see instant results; however, this route is far more successful than relying on a quick-fix plan. All of my clients who have permanently transformed their lives did not do it overnight or even in a week. Most take six to twelve months to study and master their habits. Success comes from diligently adding small new habits into your daily living.

In order to stay committed along the way, it is so important to remember your "why." Change isn't easy, so when you're faced with moments of decision, your "why" will help keep you on track. Weight loss just isn't enough. Why do you want to lose weight, get healthier, or be more mindful? Dig deep. Instead of relying on willpower for change, use your "why-power." List one to three of the most important things in your life that will drive your "why."

My Why-Power

1. _____

2. _____

3. _____

Mastering mindfulness isn't about going through periods of being perfect or failing miserably; it will be a journey full of progress and mistakes that are nothing short of valuable learning experiences. Most people fail to make permanent changes because they are discouraged when they make a mistake; they give up. They expect perfection, but instead they get the more realistic bumpy road that isn't so perfect. We have this idea in our head that people who are great were born great. However, we don't see the daily discipline of practice that led to their greatness.

Athletes don't make it to an elite level without diligent daily training. Whether or not they feel like getting out of bed, they stay committed to mastering their practice and get up anyway. If they make huge, career-risking mistakes, they get back up and keep trying. Successful business owners don't just wake up successful, either. They are dedicated to learning the complex nature of what internal and external forces influence the company's outcomes. The business that takes the time to understand these influences and quickly adapts is the one that succeeds. The business that ignores the deeper problems, resists change, and keeps trying the same patterns that aren't working will most likely fail.

So, if you find that creating change is difficult, remember that it is all a part of the process of mastering your "self." You just need to keep training. Those who are great have the courage to keep pursuing their vision when faced with struggles. Long-term change requires practice and repetition. Having a single healthy meal or a single unhealthy meal might not make much of an impact on your life. What you choose to repeatedly do will shape your habits and who you become. A child might fall fifty times before they learn to walk, but they never think, "Maybe walking isn't for me." Just keep practicing. ☺

Part 1

Exploring Your Past

"THE PAST CAN HURT, BUT YOU CAN EITHER RUN FROM IT,
OR LEARN FROM IT."
- RAFIKI, THE LION KING

The intention of this chapter is to understand the significant role your past can have in creating your habits today by exploring your level of mindfulness growing up. At the end of each section, you will be using the space provided to write your thoughts and start your path of self-discovery. The space is for you to write freely without judgment. You may use as many or as few of the lines provided as you would like. Please do not skip these very important steps that are prompted throughout this chapter. All of the information that you compile from **Part 1: Exploring the Past** and **Part 2: Observing the Present** will come together full circle and be used for **Part 3: Planning for the Future**.

Is All This Exploring Actually Important?

Regardless of what healthy eating style is chosen, most people expect that a structured meal plan and accountability will be their solution to change. Instead of reaching their goals, they will continuously reach disappointment and frustration, and having a lack of willpower usually will be to blame. We have to dig deep to understand the root of where our habits were created.

Let's be honest. At some point throughout life we have all been through some shit. But painful life lessons can be such a gift because when you're struggling and it hurts, you know you're personally growing. Life is kind of like exercising. It hurts at the time, but you have to break down the muscle before you can rebuild and grow stronger in the long run. Ideally, you should struggle, learn, grow, and be better. Unfortunately, some of those life difficulties never flourish into positive learning lessons. Instead of releasing the pain and seeing the positive, the pain becomes internalized. As more experiences come our way, we add it to the rest and suppress it, then add a little more and suppress it again. We are forced to carry the pain of our past and use distractions so we don't have to feel the uncomfortable emotions associated with the experience.

Resentment, fear, shame, self-doubt, and other emotions created as far back as childhood become a part of who we are. When a familiar situation arises, those internal feelings are triggered and we react in the same way we once did. When we have emotions or reactions to people and situations, we have to dig to the root of our suffering. The environment does not cause negative emotions and self-sabotaging behaviors. They come from within. When someone hurts our feelings or makes us mad we have to question, "Why did that bother me?" We can usually trace a trigger back to a past experience or memory.

During a conversation with a friend, I found myself being very indecisive over a simple decision. Out of a little impatience and frustration my friend said, "Quit being a people pleaser and make a decision already!" Ouch. It felt like a knife to my heart. I reacted with anger and tears in my eyes. I don't remember what I said to him, but I made it clear to never say those words to me again. I was convinced the argument was not my fault; he should have never said those hurtful words!

After a while, I started to question...why? Why did those words create pain? I knew that he cared about me and didn't intend to cause me such pain. It wasn't the words; it was the deep-rooted emotional attachment I had to the words, and I started to explore where they came from. I thought back to being a child, cleaning my sister's bedroom for her just so she would stay out of trouble. I thought back to being a teen and cleaning the kitchen just to see my mom happy about it and receive validation that I was a "good kid." I thought back to the anxious feelings I had in middle school when I hoped my friends would like me.

Maybe being a "people pleaser" isn't the worst thing to be called, but growing up that way made me unable to make decisions for myself and left me confused about my identity. I realized it was a problem when I didn't even know what I liked or didn't like anymore because every decision was based on someone else's happiness. It has been an embarrassing personality trait that I have tried to hide from other people. My suffering wasn't from the words; it was a trigger from my past that I was trying to outgrow. That self-awareness enabled me to personally change and free myself from that pain, instead of using anger, blame, or indulgences to mask and numb its roots.

If emotions, experiences, or negative thoughts are suppressed and build up, they become an integrated piece of who we are. Over time, the emotional burden that we carry becomes daily internal stress. This chronic state of stress activates the neuroendocrine system (your neurons and hormones that control the functions in your body). This triggers inflammatory and immune responses and causes the muscles to tense up as a survival mechanism. The body shifts from an anabolic "build and repair" to a catabolic "wear and tear" state. This stress becomes expressed as symptoms, such as headaches and migraines, chronic fatigue, tightness and back pain, irritability, and digestive troubles or irritable bowel syndrome (IBS). This chronic impact on our neurobiological, metabolic, and immune system is a significant contributor to age-related diseases. You can see how quickly an emotion can physically affect you if you've ever been nervous and felt the "butterflies" in your stomach. Unfortunately, most will accept their unexplainable symptoms as a part of life and eventually mask them with medications. The more we choose to accept and suppress, the more it becomes who we are, and change becomes challenging.

Uncovering and releasing those suppressed feelings gives you the ability to recreate how you respond to challenges in the future. If you keep it suppressed, it will stay a part of who you are, and history will most likely repeat itself when you are faced with familiar triggers, personal conflicts, or food decisions. Know that all of your experiences, good and bad, create who you are and are expressed through your daily habits. So you may have a lot you want to let go of, or you may just want to explore what your habits are and how you created them. Either way, understanding your past is very important to becoming more self-aware and taking control of your future.

Life would be much easier if I could just forget the years of diet mistakes I had made, the embarrassing failures with clients that I had, and experiences that I'd much rather hide from than accept. But having an honest look at my past has allowed me to change my thoughts and actions to keep history from repeating. Now, I am free to reshape my future.

I'll admit it... my past relationship with food sure wasn't

perfect. For as long as I can remember, I went on and off fad diets. I was addicted to the excitement and rush of starting something new, to be the healthiest I could be. I remember being sixteen years old, preparing for my spring break vacation, and eating popular "diet bars" because they said "healthy" across the label. Every vacation, holiday, or event had a restrictive "preparation period," followed by splurging when the date finally arrived because I "deserved it." I frequently went through the on-and-off cycles of trying low carbs, calorie counting, lemon juice concoction fasts, food combining – the list goes on. I always started off excited and ready for a "new beginning," but after a few days or a week, life's temptations crept back in and I returned to eating the same as before, if not worse. The more restrictive my diet got, the more I indulged during the rebound time. Life started becoming periods of eating perfectly or failing miserably. The push-and-pull turned food from my fuel to my enemy. Every day became "me versus food," and a daily battle for who would win. I felt like my food was taking me on a roller coaster ride that I couldn't get off of.

While I had the good intention of just trying to be healthy, I realized that the food battles were giving me an unhealthy relationship with food and had the potential to be ingrained in me for life. Between all the nutrition advice from books, magazines, websites, friends, and self-taught "health experts," I was consumed with the frustration of conflicting information, so I decided to learn the truth. I went to college and enrolled in one of the top dietetics programs in the country to become a registered dietitian. I was eager to find answers to the popularly debated question, "What's the best way to get healthy?"

After five intense years of college, I became a registered dietitian. My knowledge base was large but still unsatiated, so I continued for an additional two years to earn a master's degree in human nutrition. I now had expertise in knowing how nutrients are digested and the physiology of weight loss. My thinking was aligned with the simplified version that:

- Calories in equal to calories burned means weight maintenance.
- Fewer calories in than burned means weight loss.
- More calories in than burned means weight gain.

When I started counseling my clients, I figured that all they needed was a list of healthy foods and calorie counting for accountability so that they wouldn't overeat. I thought it was a foolproof equation to helping them, but they failed! All of them! I was baffled. It must be their lack of "willpower" because, in theory, if they're making healthy choices and eating within their calorie limits as I told them to, they would just reach their goals! But instead of achieving their goals, they reached disappointment and frustration.

Maybe it wasn't them; maybe it was me. I continued to dig to try to understand fully – why can't we reach our goals and maintain them for life? I went to conferences and seminars and reviewed research, but what I learned from the most was my own clients. When they were experiencing difficult or emotional periods in their life, they struggled with their nutrition goals, too. I became their cheerleader, helping them learn how to fuel with food instead of stressing about counting calories and measuring portions perfectly. I told them they needed to practice disconnecting their life stress from the way they ate. It was fairly solid advice.

I was really starting to help them and watch them change when life personally hit me like a sudden train wreck. I walked away from my thriving wellness company because the relationship with my business partner had gone south. My heart, soul, and savings were put into that business, but it was emotionally breaking me. I walked away from it about two weeks after my parents each invested a few thousand dollars into it with the hope of me succeeding. They were so supportive; I felt like a failure.

Within the same month, my sister/best friend moved across the country with her new best friend she met during that time. Losing both my business that I was passionate about and the closest person in my life left me empty. I continued down that path and, in the same month, I decided to end a relationship with my boyfriend of three years. He deserved to be happy, but being so heartbroken over my own life, I selfishly broke his heart, too. I felt terribly guilty, but I had no love to give to myself, let alone another person. I left the condo we were renting and embarrassingly moved back into my dad's place, where I should only have been living as a teen. For months, the loss of my "identity" and fear of the future consumed me. I didn't have a job anymore, except for the few clients who were still counseling with me, and I watched my savings drain like a ticking time bomb.

In a desperate, anxiety-driven attempt to move forward, I quickly made decisions for new business ventures, but deep inside I was full of self-doubt. My lack of confidence made me retreat from my impulsive decisions as quickly as I had gotten into them. These costly mistakes kept fueling my feelings of inadequacy and shaped the perception of who I thought I was. The belief created from my past mistakes and fear of failing in the future left me paralyzed in the present. My emotions tightened my stomach daily. I wasn't eating, but the stress was eating me alive. I was so depressed about my situation that I lost the routine, mojo, and love I had for being healthy and taking care of myself.

I remembered all the times that some of my clients had personally struggled, and my compassionate advice was "Try to get a little exercise; it will help you feel better. Activity and eating healthy can do wonders to help boost your mood!" They tried to explain that life's challenges were too overwhelming at that time to stay motivated. I judgmentally thought it was an excuse to keep putting off the work they had to do in order to accomplish their goals. Little did I know that one day I would be in their "shoes" – unable to listen to my own advice and take care of myself.

In an effort to save my health expert identity, I bought fresh fruits and vegetables, but I let them turn moldy and soggy in the fridge, only to meet their sad fate in the garbage. I used to love the complex flavors of food but everything tasted bland and boring. I went to the gym, but I stared at the weights, thought about life for ten minutes, then turned around and left. I never picked up the weights once. I would wake up exhausted and filled with negativity and go to bed with my mind racing and filled with worry. During the day, I always made sure that there were people in my presence to try to distract me from the thoughts in my head and the reality of my situation. On some evenings, a cocktail helped, too. My lifelong passions for food, cooking, and any activity were completely gone. I even started to question if I ever actually cared about being healthy, or if it was nothing but a brand I had created for myself since childhood. I still had a handful of clients who were working with me, but meeting them made me feel nervous and incompetent, and I'm sure they sensed it. How could I help them thrive if I couldn't even do it on my own?

As I began to reassemble the pieces of my life and find new outlets for happiness, my love for food and activity slowly started to creep back in. I didn't jump right back to being my "old self," but I became more self-aware and started actually using my senses again. I remember going for a walk outside and feeling the sun on my face. For the first time in months, I appreciated the sun's warmth and felt unfamiliar feelings of happiness. I remember biting into a piece of beautifully golden brown toast topped with tender avocado slices and an egg that probably wasn't perfectly cooked, but to me tasted like perfection. I finally appreciated the taste of food again. I went for long quiet drives and appreciated that I could non-judgmentally explore my thoughts or just enjoy the moment without using music as a distraction. Instead of focusing on the people who had left my life, I deeply appreciated the support I had from some of the most unexpected people. I started to be able to breathe through emotional challenges and appreciated that I could let them pass through me without consuming me. I set free the feelings I had about my past failures by realizing that they were just expensive learning experiences and didn't define who I was. At any moment, I could take the step forward to change. I surrendered to my fear of the future and chose to embrace the unknown ahead.

Alan Watts said, "The past doesn't exist. The future doesn't exist. There is only the present and that's the real you that there is." The anxiety I had created was entirely based on the past and future, neither of which is technically "real." I drew my awareness into the present and was grateful for what I had instead of what my life was lacking. I shifted my mindset from viewing myself pathetically jobless to seeing the world as full of opportunity in any direction I wished to explore. Being present allowed me to become more self-aware and tune into what I needed in that moment. I didn't do the set workout program that I was "supposed" to do; I did what felt good to my body and honored that. I explored what habits drained my energy and positive spirit and which ones inspired and energized me. I've never been the person to end a day with "Dear Diary," but journaling became the key to seeing the "aha" moments about myself that were life-changing. Once I let go of my frustrations about the past and worries for my future, I discovered how to be present, happy, and healthy again.

Going through that difficult time made me truly realize that emotions and past experiences are strongly connected to the way we eat, how we handle stress, how much stress we actually allow in our lives, and our perception of what we believe we are capable of today. It sure wasn't a fun experience, but I learned more about myself and my habits than I ever have. When I saw my clients struggle, I no longer just had strategies to help them; I really understood them. The more they explored their past and their present situations and feelings, the more self-aware they became. I didn't have solutions to their problems, but the more they were willing to explore, the better they saw their relationship to food and triggers that continually sabotaged their goals. Instead of eating perfectly when life was easy and quitting when life was tough, they saw why they struggled and kept persevering. Through patience, self-discovery, and reconnecting with their bodies, my clients were succeeding... every single one of them.

Everyone develops their own personal relationship to food, which is why self-discovery is essential. There are many different scenarios in life that can influence our eating. Take a look at some of these examples:

Infancy: When the mother is breastfeeding and the baby pulls its head away, the nurturing mother typically brings the baby's mouth to the nipple to resume feeding. While the mother is only trying to make sure the baby is well fed, this sends the very first message of: "Ignore your feelings of satisfaction; mom will tell you how much to eat."

Baby: When a crying baby is given a pacifier, a soothing and comforting oral fixation is created.

Toddler and Childhood: At this stubborn age, they're often told not to leave the table until the plate is finished. This rule teaches them to use their plate to guide how much they should eat, instead of tuning into their hunger and satiety signals. Snacks and treats are given as a reward for good behavior, which creates an unnatural attachment to food and treats. When they are "bad" and treats are withheld, a void is created and the good feeling that food brought them is taken away. When treats were once given, then later not allowed, some children will start sneaking and hiding food. This unhealthy relationship to food can continue for a lifetime.

Teen: With emotions raging at this age, teenagers often find comfort in food to soothe boredom while watching TV, relieve heartaches from dating, or to celebrate winning at a sport. This vulnerable age can establish the emotional connection to food that can also endure through adulthood.

Adulthood: After a long, stressful day, many people just want to come home to crunchy, salty snacks and a glass of wine to unwind after a long day of work.

One of my earliest food memories as a child was not being able to sleep late at night, so my dad would let me stroll down to the kitchen with him. He let me sit on the counter and have an ice cream sandwich. It was a good memory and makes me smile when I think about it today. For years after, ice cream became our "thing" between my dad and me. No one else in the family really cared for ice cream, so it was our special time for a late trip to the store to pick up our favorite flavors before a movie night. I decided to stop eating dairy a long time ago for health reasons, but if I hadn't, would I have found comfort in ice cream today from those memories? Maybe, but maybe not. If ice cream was a part of my diet today, it would be important to observe whether it is an occasional treat or a comforting food that I struggle to have control over.

Certain environmental cues today can trigger a pleasurable or mealtime memory from the past and lead to a craving. Remember those food slogans and ad campaigns? Here's one from Little Debbie: "It's a fact: you never outgrow your love for Little Debbie snacks." Don't underestimate how the foods from your past can influence your food choices now. Understanding your past can help you see how your present habits have been created, and how you can deal with unresolved issues that may be sabotaging your goals.

Maria was an extremely fast eater. She often scarfed her food so fast that, on several occasions, she swallowed her food whole and almost choked. Food became a problem for her because she wasn't experiencing the taste of her food and couldn't pay attention to how hungry she was along the way. This left her unsatisfied but stuffed after eating.

When she started questioning her fast eating habits, she looked into her past. She remembered that her anxious mom made eating time very rushed, always pressuring her to finish up her plate because they were already late for the day's events. She also thought back to the many years she had worked in the restaurant industry. Break time was so short that she was constantly rushed to mow down some food before getting back to work.

Once she became aware of her eating behaviors from her past, she was able to set up boundaries between herself and memories of her anxious mom, and remind herself that she no longer worked at the restaurant. From then on, she was able to recognize when she started to rush and practiced slowing down and listening to her hunger cues to regain control over her food and enjoy the experience of eating.

Let's take a closer look into your past to see how it may be influencing your habits today. You may be thinking, "But I don't have any bad memories from my past!" Most of us have had plenty of experiences that shaped who we are; you may just need to do a little digging. Your experiences may be full of struggle and challenges, positive and happy moments, or perhaps neither good nor bad but valuable enough to observe and explore. The more thorough you are uncovering your past, the better you can understand your habits today and create effective solutions for changing your future. If you haven't spent much time thinking about your past, try to stay open-minded and give yourself a little time to dig. Know that the purpose of this section is to deepen your self-exploration and is not a replacement for psychological counseling or professional help.

Mindful Eating: What Are Your Food Memories?

Past memories can help you see how your relationship with food was created. Many eating habits are a learned behavior, so it is good to go back and explore the roots of what presently influences your eating. Your initial thought might be that you don't have any specific food memories but most find that when they spend time thinking about their past they uncover many. You could even gain further insight by asking your family members about their perspectives and memories from your family traditions. I come from an Italian family, so my grandfather would make homemade pasta every Sunday. This tradition brought my family together and created so many of our happy memories. Since my grandfather passed away, people in my family often talk about the comforting feeling that eating pasta brings.

Try to recall any scenarios in your past that involved food. These memories might be positive, comforting, and celebratory, or they might be negative and even painful. Here are a few questions to get you thinking:

- Did your parents tell you to finish what was on your plate?
- Did you feel guilty or "bad" for eating certain foods?
- Did you feel like you had to sneak certain foods?
- Do you have a happy memory about one specific food?
- Did your family or friends encourage fad diets?
- Did you have to eat all of your food out of guilt for other people in starving countries?
- Does your family have certain eating or food traditions?
- Did you eat certain foods only because you didn't want to hurt the cook's feelings?

- Did you have one particular favorite food for certain celebrations, such as winning a team sport or going out for a birthday celebration?

Give yourself the time and freedom to explore fully your past relationship with food in order to bring awareness to your habits today. This is an important step in the process so don't skip it! The thoughts you come up with will help you see your habits more clearly when you move on to Part 2: Observing the Present. Write your memories in this section. If you need more space to write, additional sheets can be downloaded from:

www.Gina-B.com/MindfulnessMastery

Exploring the Past: Mindful Eating

Based on the memories you came up with, how do you relate to those foods or situations today? Start noticing if you have kept your past rules, traditions, or food choices in your lifestyle today. When you better understand how your habits were created in the past, you can become empowered to reshape your future.

Mindful Living: Where Have You Struggled?

Throughout life we will all be presented with challenges and emotional burdens. Maybe it was the loss of a friend or family member, a breakup or divorce, losing a job or passion you loved, taking emotional or physical abuse from a toxic relationship, or some experience that left a lasting personal scar. You may have found ways to resolve or make peace with those challenges; sometimes, however, when they're too much to bear, they become suppressed. By not facing difficult emotions or experiences, it's easy to use food or other pleasures to keep from thinking about or reliving the pain.

Research Review: The cost of suppressing stressful memories

A study by Klein and Bratton explored the effects of suppressed memories on adult cognitive performance. Results showed that exploring unwanted thoughts actually competes for cognitive reserves, which has an effect on performing mental tasks. Attempts to suppress unwanted thoughts can be a cause for depression, mood disorders, and other psychological issues.

Understanding and dealing with difficult situations are essential to releasing suppressed pain and to create mental and emotional space for happiness.

Charlene had been working one-on-one with me for about ten months to make healthier choices and practice better portion control to result in weight loss. Charlene continually kept hitting a roadblock. "Why do I always sabotage myself?" she'd ask. "I do so well; I love the healthy food I'm eating. I feel great and then BAM! Cravings attack and take over. I can't stop them!"

Charlene took a few days for self-discovery. She honestly and non-judgmentally wrote down any thoughts, feelings, and eating experiences she had. It didn't take long for her to realize that past deaths in her family were difficult for her to deal with, and she'd never made peace with them. When her emotions began to creep in, she noticed her urge to grab snacks to create a comforting distraction from the pain.

Once she recognized this pattern, she found new ways to cope with the painful memories instead of keeping them suppressed with food. She accepts that sometimes it might be painful to experience the feelings, but she learns that it is a normal part of grieving and doesn't always have to be suppressed or resolved. Charlene admits that it isn't always easy, but she's made leaps and bounds in regaining control over her food.

Exploring unresolved feelings or situations is a key piece in healing the relationship with yourself and being free from using food to cope. You can't create a new future if you keep holding onto habits of the past. Some find that their personality traits from childhood, such as anxiety, stress, or having a temper, continue into adulthood and trigger bad habits, such as over-eating, using alcohol or drugs, or starting arguments with others. Exploring your past doesn't mean that you have to change your personality traits or accept situations that caused personal pain. What it can do is help you predict a situation that might create emotions, such as frustration, sadness, anger, fear, or anxiety. You can then find an effective outlet to handle those emotions rather than keeping them suppressed and internalized or acting out irrationally.

Think about what memories make you feel uncomfortable, angry, or sad and use this as an opportunity to see what emotions you are still holding onto.

Here are a few questions to provoke your thoughts:

- What personality traits do people who know you say that you have?
- How did you handle stress growing up?
- How did you respond to difficult situations?
- What were the most challenging life moments in your past?

This could be anytime from childhood to yesterday. It might be a personality trait, habit, or a difficult situation or experience, such as a bad relationship with your family or a significant other, a death, or an illness. Use this section to explore anything you need to better understand or set yourself free from your past. Dig deep, and write about anything you may have suppressed. Again, additional sheets are available at:

www.Gina-B.com/MindfulnessMastery.

Exploring the Past: Mindful Living

Mindful Self-Talk:
What Was Your Self-Perception?

Your self-perception as you were growing up can have a significant influence on how you talk to yourself today. Negative thoughts will always sabotage your health goals and overall outlook on life. Our mind is very powerful; our actions will follow any thoughts or beliefs that we have about ourselves to keep us as that same comfortable person. Profound change comes from a mindset shift in who we believe we are and in what we can accomplish.

Those who were hard on themselves in their younger years often continue with similar self-talk into adulthood. Your own thoughts or someone else's could have created the belief about who you are entirely. Bold statements and remarks could come from your parents, friends, teachers, athletic coaches, or even strangers. Sometimes we don't even realize that we allowed their comments to enter in as a part of our identity.

Heather shared a memory of her past. She painfully retold the story... "When I would go over to my friend's house, her mom would call me Heifer, instead of Heather. I was only twelve years old. It left a big impact on me when I was younger and I'll never forget it."

Heather has spent years dedicated to personal growth studies to become aware of her own self-talk and the impact it leaves.

Heather reminds herself that she is a strong, beautiful woman, which allows her to exude that description, and not the "heifer" that someone tried to identify her as.

Think about the timeline of your life and who has influenced the way that you perceive yourself. Learning to be kind to yourself, which we will focus on later, is a key part in ending the Destructive Self-Sabotaging Cycle. Here are a few questions to consider:

- What did you think of yourself as a kid, as a teen, and as a young adult?
- Were you happy with your physical appearance and abilities?
- How do you think other people thought of you? How did you talk to yourself?
- Do you still say some of those same things today?

These questions are meant to help you explore your memories. Use as much of the space as you would like in this section or download additional pages from:

www.Gina-B.com/MindfulnessMastery.

Exploring the Past: Mindful Self-Talk

The Power of Positivity

When you are setting new goals and making changes, the mind has a tendency to focus on what has not yet been accomplished, instead of what has. This perpetuates the cycle of disappointment, low self-esteem, and feelings of inadequacy during a journey that is expected to have challenges and learning lessons. When accomplishments so small become naturally integrated into the lifestyle, they tend to get overlooked. When each "win" is praised, you are acknowledging the positive accomplishment to keep driving forward your change versus feeling disappointed and inadequate from what you are still working on.

Next, write five personal accomplishments for which you are proud. Your list may or may not be health related. Accomplishments could be leaving an unfulfilling job, a job achievement, raising your kids, quitting smoking, going back to or finishing school, having the courage to make a big life change, eating vegetables that you never thought you would try, creating a new habit that positively impacted your life, *etc.*

My Accomplishments

1. _____
2. _____
3. _____
4. _____
5. _____

Summary

When we heal and release the stories or beliefs we have created about ourselves from the past, we can begin to create a new future that doesn't repeat itself. Based on what you wrote, think about which pieces of your past may be influencing your life today. You may see a clearer picture when you move to the next section: Observing the Present. For now, make a mental note of which past feelings or experiences you can make peace with and release. Also, think about which ones you should face and deal with, so you don't keep them suppressed. It's time to take those emotions that are being stored in your subconscious mind and body and set them free so you can finally create a new future. Any fear, disappointments, resentment, worry, or anger will no longer serve your purpose in change.

I understand that the thought of facing and releasing what you have suppressed may sound like an undesirable task, but holding onto it will only cause you to retain physical and/or emotional stress and repeat behaviors in the future. You may feel the need to confront a past situation or seek help from a therapist to resolve suppressed feelings, as this book is not intended to replace any needed psychological counseling. Digging through your past will help you identify which foods, scenarios, or thoughts are triggers or coping mechanisms for you during difficult situations. We will discuss triggers later in the book and use this list to create an effective plan. Let go of any fear you have moving forward and embrace your exploratory journey ahead.

Part 2

Observing the Present

> "SELF-AWARENESS IS HAVING THE ABILITY TO TAKE AN HONEST LOOK AT YOUR LIFE WITHOUT HAVING ANY ATTACHMENT TO IT BEING RIGHT OR WRONG, GOOD OR BAD."
>
> – DEBBIE FORD

Now that you've explored the past, you'll have an opportunity to closely observe your present day-to-day life in order to see how your eating, everyday habits, and thoughts all influence each other. No change or plan of action is needed here; the entire purpose is to observe and learn without judgment. Think of it as being your own researcher to really understand what is going on. Try to let go of any embarrassment or shame for mistakes that you make. These moments will give you the most valuable insights to better understand your patterns and triggers and to empower you to make a change. You can't change what you are not aware of. An interpretation of your observations with solutions will come later, as I don't want it to influence your current habits. The more honest you are with yourself, the better you can understand where you struggle. This will help you make a clear plan in Part 3 to make changes successfully.

Mindful Eating

Without changing your current eating habits, keep a seven-day food log using the charts in this section. It's very important that you keep to your typical diet and commit to logging during this time. I don't recommend long-term rigid food logging, but try to commit to at least seven days so you can really understand your eating habits. Seven days of logging will allow you to see the full picture of how you eat throughout the week. Your habits on Monday may be drastically different from your habits on Saturday. A few days might give you some insight, but you could be missing the whole picture! It may seem like a lot of work, but the food log is relatively simple, and completing this step is critical to discovering where you struggle. Include days that you'd call "the good, the bad, and the ugly." Try to refrain from measuring perfect portions or calorie counting, as this activity is purely observational. This log is not accountability for sticking to a healthy diet. I recommend filling out your form as you eat throughout the day, or immediately after, instead of relying on your memory at the end of the day. There are more than seven charts available in case you need additional space for one day. Once you have the seven-day record filled out, we will break down what it all means. If you'd like to record your eating habits for more than seven days, additional sheets are available at *www.Gina-B.com/MindfulnessMastery*. Be kind to yourself and try not to judge as you observe your habits. Over time, they'll improve. Have patience.

At this time, spend the next seven days filling out the food log before reading any further. I don't recommend reading ahead while you are logging because the explanations may influence your way of eating. Observing your natural way of eating is critical to understand where you personally struggle. The first chart is an example of how to fill out the log. It is not a sample meal plan or guide.

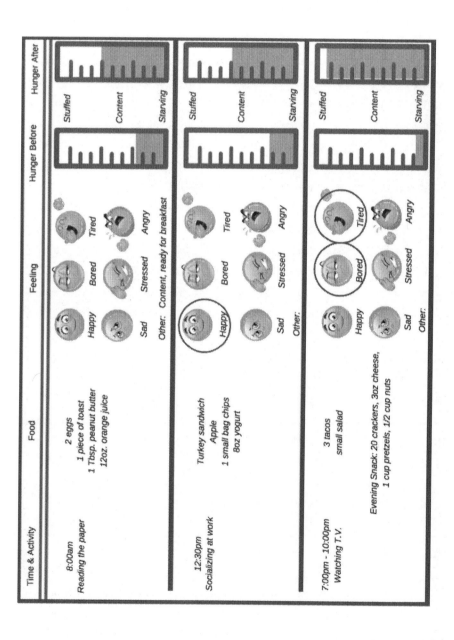

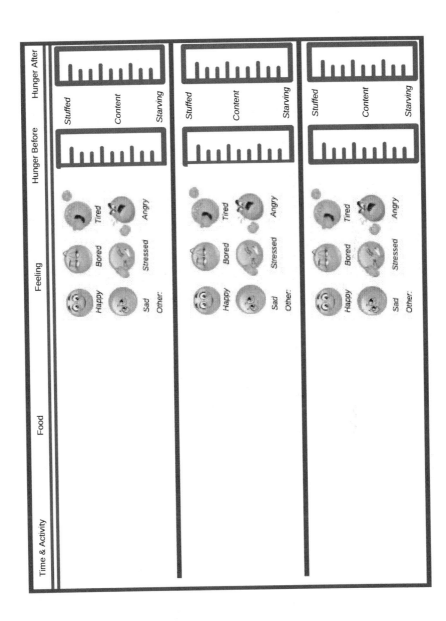

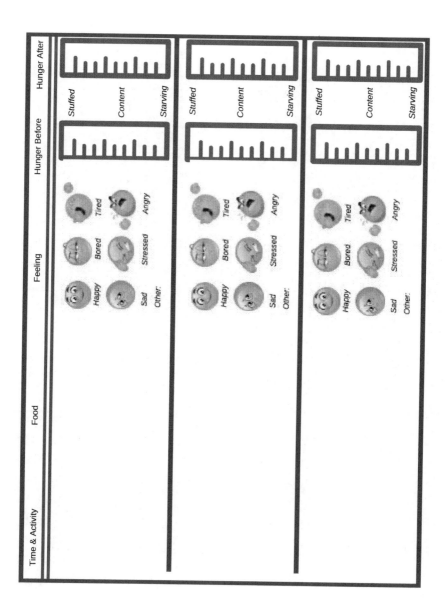

Time & Activity	Food	Feeling	Hunger Before	Hunger After
		Happy Bored Tired Sad Stressed Angry Other:	Stuffed — Content — Starving	Stuffed — Content — Starving
		Happy Bored Tired Sad Stressed Angry Other:	Stuffed — Content — Starving	Stuffed — Content — Starving
		Happy Bored Tired Sad Stressed Angry Other:	Stuffed — Content — Starving	Stuffed — Content — Starving

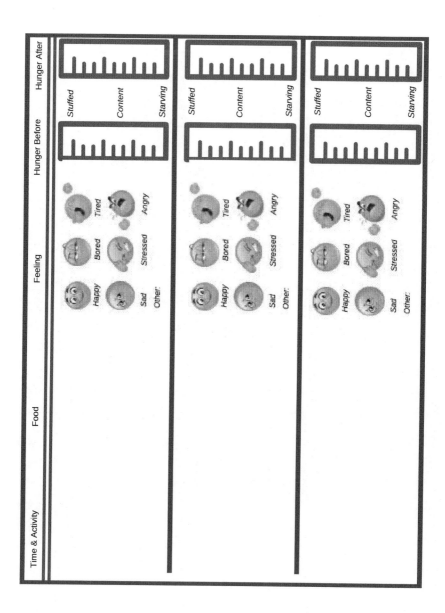

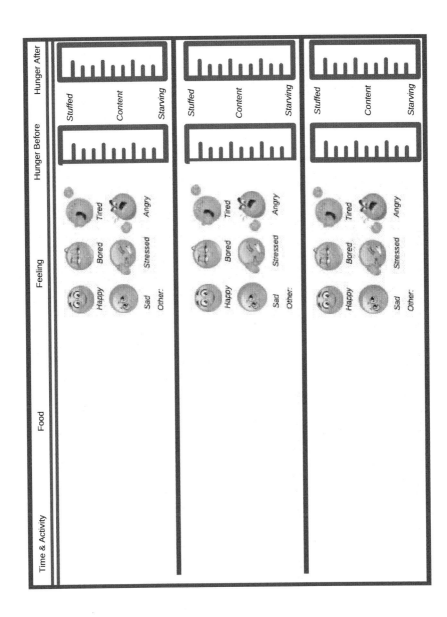

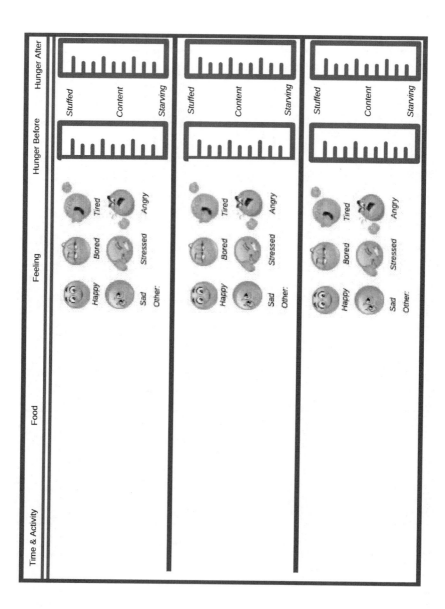

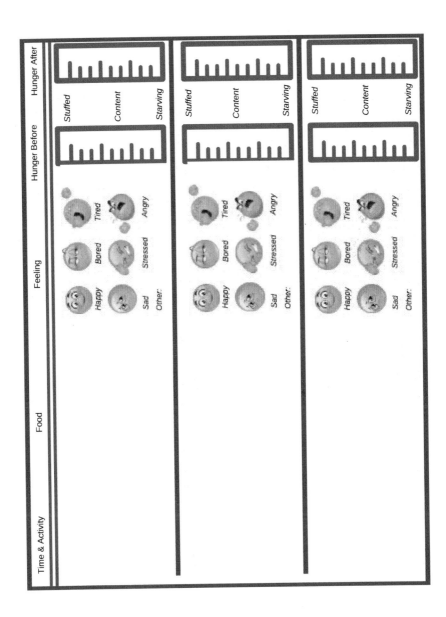

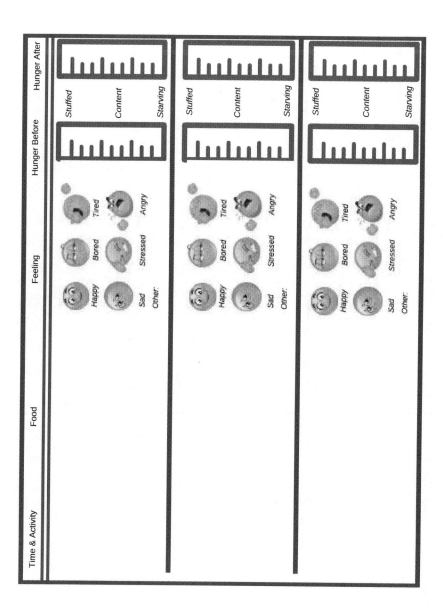

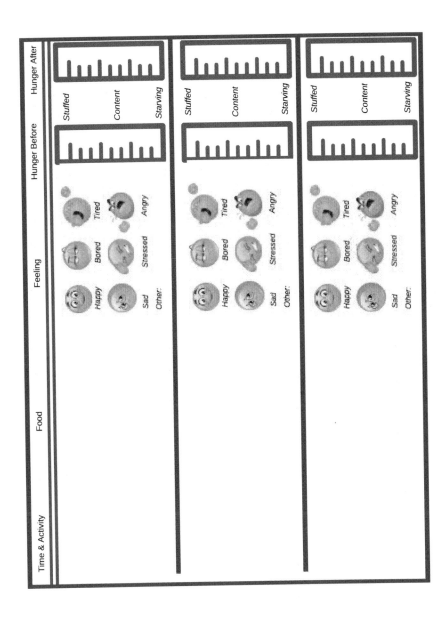

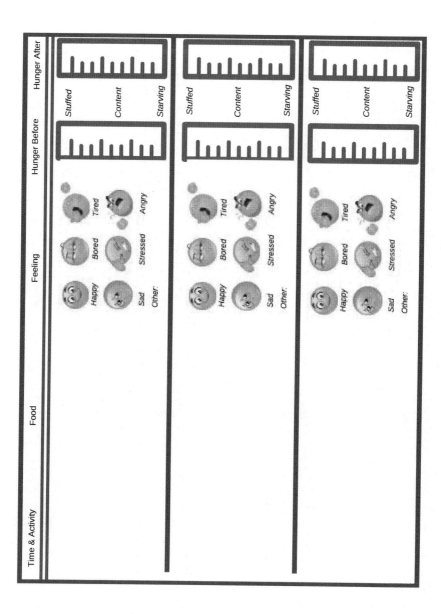

Time & Activity	Food	Feeling	Hunger Before	Hunger After
		Tired Angry Bored Stressed Happy Sad Other:	|..|..|..|..| Stuffed — Content — Starving	|..|..|..|..| Stuffed — Content — Starving
		Tired Angry Bored Stressed Happy Sad Other:	|..|..|..|..| Stuffed — Content — Starving	|..|..|..|..| Stuffed — Content — Starving
		Tired Angry Bored Stressed Happy Sad Other:	|..|..|..|..| Stuffed — Content — Starving	|..|..|..|..| Stuffed — Content — Starving

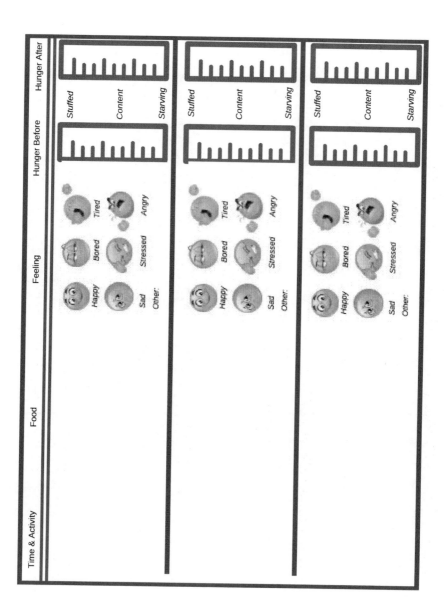

Time & Activity	Food	Feeling	Hunger Before	Hunger After
		Tired Angry Bored Stressed Happy Sad Other:	Stuffed / Content / Starving	Stuffed / Content / Starving
		Tired Angry Bored Stressed Happy Sad Other:	Stuffed / Content / Starving	Stuffed / Content / Starving
		Tired Angry Bored Stressed Happy Sad Other:	Stuffed / Content / Starving	Stuffed / Content / Starving

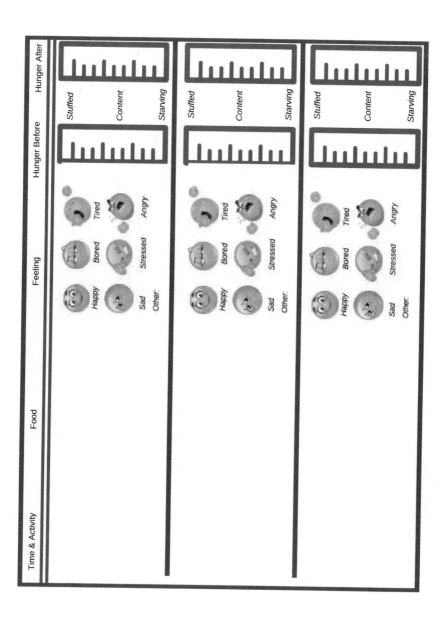

What Did You Learn?

After each topic below, summarize what you learned about each part of the Food Log. This part is very important and will be used to create your customized *Mindfulness Mastery Plan* in Part 3 where we will further interpret your findings and customize solutions to your struggles. No plan of action is needed here. The purpose is to observe any patterns or habits that you have.

Time: Were your eating times (e.g., breakfast, lunch, and dinner) fairly regular throughout the day, or did they vary? Were there times when you went without eating for a long period of time or did you find that you were eating often, more like grazing?

_____
_____
_____
_____
_____
_____
_____
_____

Large gaps without eating are likely to cause overeating later. You may need to practice eating at regular intervals to help balance your meal portions throughout the day. If you're eating too often, it could mean that you're eating for other reasons, which we'll address later.

Food: Were you happy with the food choices you made? Did you find any patterns of having healthier balanced meals at certain times, and less healthy choices such as cookies, chips, or candy at other times? What food choices would you like to change?

_____
_____
_____
_____

This information can tell you if you're happy with the way you're currently eating, and when you're the most vulnerable to the less healthy food temptations. If you noticed that your food choices were poor around certain times of the day, or in certain situations, this can tell you what triggers you to eat these foods. You might even be able to tell what foods trigger you to overeat. If certain foods make you feel out of control and lead to overeating, you may want to avoid them during your mindful eating practice that we will start using in Part 3. They don't necessarily have to be eliminated forever, but at least until you feel confident and in control when eating. I know that having complete control over indulgences may sound as likely as riding a unicorn, but be patient and trust the process and you will get there.

Quantity: What did you notice about how much food you ate? Did the amount gradually increase, decrease, or stay the same throughout the day? Summarize your quantities of food throughout the day from your food journal and note any patterns or trends.

If the amount of food gradually increased throughout the day, it's likely that you're not eating enough food earlier, which causes you to overeat in the evening. Meals or snacks that are larger than what you would normally eat may let you know that something is causing you to overeat in a certain situation.

Hunger: What did you notice about your hunger level? Did it correlate to the quantity of food you ate, your food choices, or what times you ate? It can be helpful to gauge your hunger level by using a scale of 1 to 10.

> <u>Hunger Level 1-2:</u> You're so hungry you feel like you're starving, shaky, and maybe even hangry (hungry + angry)! You never want to get to this level. It means you've waited too long to eat. This is what I call the Zombie Attack. The Zombie Attack happens when you let yourself get so hungry that you lose all rationality and could eat just about anything in sight. It could be a bag of chips, cookies, your cat, or your own left arm. Look out for the Zombie Attack! Most people notice that if they let themselves get to a level of 1 or 2 on the hunger scale, they'll overeat at their next meal. Long stretches without eating, or not eating enough food, can be the cause of overeating and making poor food choices.
>
> <u>Hunger Level 3-4:</u> You're slightly hungry and ready to eat. Periods of tummy rumbling may come and go signaling that food will be needed pretty soon.
>
> <u>Hunger Level 5-6</u>: You feel content and satisfied.
>
> <u>Hunger Level 7-8:</u> You feel a little too full and may have been better off without those extra bites.
>
> <u>Hunger Level 9-10:</u> You feel full to absolutely stuffed! If you notice that you're eating when your hunger level is at a 6 or higher, you'll really want to look into why you're eating (remember, 5-6 is a satisfied level). That discussion will come in Part 3.

Write any notes about your hunger levels when you were eating:

_____
_____
_____
_____
_____
_____
_____
_____
_____
_____
_____

Doing: What were you doing when you were eating? Make note if you were watching TV, working on your computer, reading, browsing through your phone, drinking with friends, driving, etc. How did this influence your food choices or how much you ate? Distractions often cause overeating because you're not paying attention to how full and satisfied you are. Summarize what you learned from the food log about what you do while you eat.

_____
_____
_____
_____
_____
_____
_____
_____
_____
_____
_____
_____

Feelings: What were you feeling when you were eating? Were there emotions or situations, such as boredom, stress, loneliness, or anxiety that triggered you to eat certain foods or quantities? Discovering your triggers will help you be aware of what causes your unhealthy eating patterns. Summarize what you learned and be sure to note any connection you see between feelings you had or situations going on and the food choices you made. In the next section, you'll create an alternate plan of action to handle those feelings without using food.

_____
_____
_____
_____
_____
_____
_____
_____
_____
_____
_____
_____
_____
_____
_____
_____
_____
_____
_____
_____
_____
_____
_____
_____
_____
_____
_____

Social Situations

Certain social situations can trigger overeating as well, such as snacking at a party, going out to eat with friends, work gatherings or lunches, and going out to the movies. When starting a new diet plan, most people want to hide at home and not engage in social happenings because they might overeat, indulge in forbidden foods, or drink too much and end up sabotaging their goals... but we can't avoid life forever!

Being prepared and practicing mindfulness is far more effective than hiding out until you finally give in at the next event or holiday. It's not that you can't eat or indulge at social gatherings, but that you do so mindfully, not mindlessly. Being aware of these situations will help you create a plan so that you stay mindful and don't sabotage your goals. What social situations, such as certain friends, work meetings, social events, or holidays, are frequently challenging for you? Write about these situations in the next space provided. In Part 3 we will go into effective strategies to help you plan for these situations.

Mindful Living: What Can You Control? What Do You Need To Let Go?

Stress puts an incredible amount of wear and tear on the body, so being aware of what triggers your stress will be key to mastering the techniques for your stress management plan in Part 3. This is the time to observe the world around you, to see how you respond to and handle challenging situations. At times, we let our external environment create significant stress that we aren't even aware of. Writing it on paper can help to see how often you let stress affect you and better evaluate which situations you should practice letting go of and which you should think about addressing. Pay close attention to what you focus your attention on and what people or situations make you angry or stressed. Notice whether they are temporary (such as a traffic jam or flight delay, dealing with an angry customer or co-worker, or waiting in a long line), or ongoing (such as financial troubles, an illness, or family or relationship problems). Include in the list what is making you stressed, angry, or unhappy, covering these components for each situation:

1. **What is the cause of the stress?**

2. **Did I impulsively react or appropriately respond to the situation?**

Before you read any further, spend one day observing the stress you encounter. Notice if you find your mind preoccupied with the past or racing into the future. In this section, write down your observations. In Part 3 we will go over how stress affects our eating habits and mental, emotional, and physical health along with the key strategies to effectively manage stress. Again, additional sheets are available at

www.Gina-B.com/MindfulnessMastery

After taking the time to observe your stress, think about what makes you happy. Do you take breaks in your busy day, or make a plan to do the things that make you happy? We aren't usually forced to sit down and think about what actually makes us happy, so take advantage of this opportunity! This could be as simple as a hot bath, a good book on a Sunday, or a quick walk outside while at work, or as big as a week's vacation in the tropics. Make a list of at least five things that make you happy and note if you are making time for them in your schedule.

1. _____
2. _____
3. _____
4. _____
5. _____
6. _____
7. _____
8. _____
9. _____
10. _____

Mindful Self-Talk: How Do You Talk To Yourself? Are You Being Nice?

We often don't realize that the voice in our head talks and talks, relaying messages all day long. Self-talk is usually at its highest when we look in the mirror and before or after eating, but it could be at any point throughout the day. It is important to be aware of what we say to ourselves, as it isn't always fully accurate or truly reflective of what we are capable of accomplishing. Being aware of your self-talk is key to gaining control over your thoughts and making a change. In Part 3 we will dig deeper into how your thoughts control your actions and patterns of behavior.

Try to explore the voice in your head throughout the day; *do not* skip this critical part! Your self-talk may be about your physical appearance, capabilities, accomplishments, habits, or skills in a positive or negative manner. Again, no change is needed here, as this is a non-judgmental, observational activity. Before reading any further, record any positive or negative words or phrases you say to yourself for at least one day. In Part 3 we will also address the key strategies to master you mind to become empowered in overcoming your self-imposed limitations.

Self-talk when I first wake up in the morning:

_____
_____
_____
_____
_____
_____
_____
_____
_____

Self-talk when I look in the mirror:

_____
_____
_____
_____
_____
_____
_____
_____
_____

Self-talk before and after eating:

_____
_____
_____
_____
_____
_____
_____
_____
_____

Other positive or negative self-talk throughout the day:

_____
_____
_____
_____
_____
_____
_____
_____

Part 3

Planning for the Future

"Failing to prepare is preparing to fail."
- Benjamin Franklin

Now that you've observed your eating habits, daily stress, what makes you happy, and how you talk to yourself, you'll be able to see clearly where you struggle. In Part 3 you will create a plan to predict situations when you're most vulnerable and implement the right strategies so you can break through any barriers to changing your life and building new habits. It will be very helpful to look back at your notes to make sure you include all the pieces of your plan to set yourself up for success.

Mindful Eating

In order to *master mindful eating,* it's critical to abstain from a typical "fad diet" mentality and instead shift the focus toward more self-awareness. Rebuilding your relationship with food and building new habits are keys to creating a long-lasting and healthier life, but they do take time and patience.

While you are practicing to eat in control and more mindfully, I don't recommend measuring perfect portions or counting calories. When you are busy calorie counting, you are ignoring your body's signals and relying on numbers instead, creating a greater disconnect from your body. Most calorie-counters admit that when they don't know the calories in a meal, they have an "ignorance is bliss" moment and end up overeating. A standard calorie-restricted diet also doesn't accurately predict how much food you actually need, how fast your metabolism is, or how much activity you have had during the day. The best way to know how much to eat is to listen to the signals that your body is sending. Eating strategies, such as choosing healthier foods that will stabilize blood sugar, planning meals and snacks, and staying hydrated, can make a big difference in listening to true hunger signals. We will dive into more nutrition strategies later. Letting go of any rules might seem scary, but slowly you will be able to intuitively listen to your body's signals and trust yourself again.

Even if your goal is to lose weight, weighing yourself can be counterproductive, at least when starting. When most people are just starting to make healthier changes and weigh themselves often, they become so focused on the number and want to give up when it doesn't change right away or if they see the numbers fluctuate. Also, if you're starting a strength-training program, you might see your weight initially increase from building muscle. You don't want those numbers to deter you from what you are accomplishing! Many people often panic when they see the scale go up after they have been working out so diligently. Once they stay consistent with their habits and notice that their clothes are fitting much looser, they're relieved. Let go of any focus on your weight and instead immerse yourself in the journey of getting there. You first need to build the foundational habits that will later result in physical changes.

Think of it like putting together a puzzle. The completed puzzle is the "bigger picture," such as weight loss or getting healthier. Each behavior change is a piece of that puzzle. If you dumped 1000 pieces in a pile and had to fit them all together at once, it would probably feel quite overwhelming. To tackle a big puzzle, most people start with the corner pieces and fill in the picture one piece at a time. Consider reading this book as your corner piece. You are taking the steps to complete your puzzle but without actually following through with actions, your puzzle will not be complete! Accomplishing small goals or changes may feel insignificant, but every time you add one, you are building a strong, beautiful, unbreakable picture.

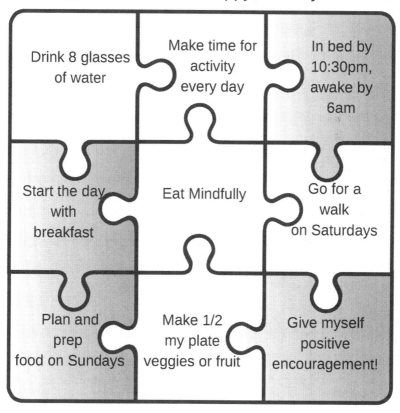

No matter how small of a change, be proud every time you add another habit to continue your momentum! Take the time to build a strong foundation before you expect to see results (your "bigger picture"). You may lose the excitement and "rush" from starting a new diet that creates instant results, but remind yourself that those diets never work long-term. It's time for a life change that is driven by your "why-power," not a quick fix that relies on your willpower. Keep reflecting on your Why-Power List that you came up with to keep driving forward your change.

The first step in practicing mindful eating is to use your hunger signals to guide how much to eat. This is a great strategy for anyone to practice to better listen to their body's needs. Children, teens, adults, and the elderly are all regularly exposed to a mindless environment and could benefit from practicing mindful eating. The weight loss industry also has instilled the idea that hunger is bad and we need to find ways to suppress our appetite. In reality, when you truly tune into your hunger signals, you will know when and how much to eat. Your true hunger signals are a sign that your body needs more fuel. Fullness is a sign that you have had enough energy. If you're used to relying on a structured meal plan, it may take time and practice using your hunger to guide your eating instead of counting or measuring.

Think back to that 1-10 scale to evaluate how hungry you actually are before eating, while you eat, and after eating. When you're a little hungry and have a slight rumble in your stomach that gradually starts to come and go, you're probably around a 3-4, which indicates a good time to eat. Think of eating like a rollercoaster. The goal is to have smaller hills to go up and down (as in the first roller coaster picture) rather than large hills (as in the second picture). The large low dips represent long periods without eating, which almost always results in a big shift toward overeating. This large change in calorie restriction to over-abundance doesn't give your body the consistent calories it needs to maintain a healthy weight.

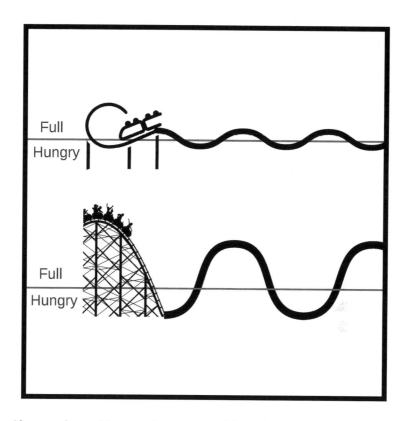

If you often skip meals, you could probably expect a big uphill of overeating heading your way. The more consistently you can eat when you start to feel hungry, the better you can give your body a steady supply of energy that it needs. Remember, the more you restrict and deprive yourself, the more you're likely to put yourself on the big rollercoaster style of eating. These large fluctuations of deprivation and overeating create internal stress on the body and can cause fatigue, intense sugar and carbohydrate cravings often leading to poor food choices, difficulty managing weight, and other health problems associated with elevated stress hormones.

Becoming in tune with your hunger will help you manage this roller coaster ride. You may have a strong urge to eat, but being aware of the different types of hunger can also help you dig deeper into understanding why you want to eat.

Physical Hunger: This type of hunger gradually builds when you haven't had food to eat for a while – typically three to five hours after your last meal. You may start to hear your stomach growling with gentle hunger pains. If you wait too long to eat, you may feel a little shaky from a drop in blood sugar. Listening to your physical hunger signals will help guide you in knowing when you physiologically need to eat.

Sensory Hunger: This type of hunger comes on almost instantly when your senses are stimulated. It could be from the sight, smell, or taste of food. It is easy to underestimate the strong influence your senses can have on driving you to eat, but it all comes back to instinct. When cavemen didn't have guidance on what to eat, their innate sensory cues helped them choose safe and nutritious foods. Attractive colors, smells, and flavors stimulated their hunger and activated the reward centers in the brain so that when appealing food was present, the natural drive to eat would continue.

Food images, especially from palatable foods, heighten neurological responses in the brain. Physiological changes then take place, such as saliva production and insulin release, to prepare the body to eat. This creates the natural drive to eat from the sight of food. However, not everyone has an equal response to food images. Very low-calorie dieters have a stronger response to the sight of food. In one study, eighty-five female participants were shown visual images of chocolate. After viewing the images, those on a restrictive diet scored significantly higher than non-dieters on questionnaires that evaluated the desire for certain foods. The study concluded that food images increase cravings, especially for dieters avoiding "forbidden" foods, and may induce guilt, anxiety, and depression. So be aware that the more restrictive your diet is, the more likely you will desire the foods you are trying to not eat.

The physiological changes that happen from the sight of food have been the foundation for chefs to create enticing meals based on the concept that people "eat with their eyes." From celebrity chefs and cooking channels, to Instagram and other social media, the "food porn" industry is enticing us to eat more than ever before. Photos now capture so much detail of steam and texture that you could almost taste it just by looking. Tuning into your sensory hunger can help you become more aware of what stimuli might trigger overeating and to differentiate true physical hunger from sensory hunger.

Emotional Hunger: This type of hunger typically comes on very rapidly from a surge of emotion. Most people find these feelings very intense and refuse to wait patiently for food. They must find food NOW! These cravings for food are often used to fill an emotional void, such as loneliness, sadness, stress, or anxiety.

Being aware of the type of hunger you're experiencing will help you be mindful and will be a key piece to making your Mindfulness Mastery Plan at the end of this section. At first, you may find it difficult to differentiate the type of hunger you are experiencing. When you feel hungry, observe what description is most fitting to your current situation. Over time, you will be able to immediately know if it is physical hunger or not and practice to fulfill what you really need.

If you have assessed your hunger and you realize that you don't have the physical hunger sensations, the next step in mindful eating is to ask yourself, "Why do I want to eat?" Take a look back at your food log and your notes about what you learned. Were you usually eating because of physical hunger, sensory hunger, or emotional hunger? If you notice that you are not eating because of physical hunger, you could be using food to create a distraction or suppress a feeling. If so, it's very important to go back to your notes in Part 2: Mindful Living: What Can You Control? What Do You Need to Let Go? – to uncover what is currently bothering you. You may also want to look back to your notes in Part 1: Exploring Your Past, to see if your past feelings are being suppressed with food.

Mary spent most of her days working from home in a stressful job that required long hours of computer work. Whenever she hit a mental block and frustration, she found herself creeping into the kitchen to delay the work that needed to be done. When she started to ask herself, "What do I really need right now?" she was able to tune-in and understand herself better. Mary decided to schedule a mid-day yoga session to boost her energy and refresh her mind. She realized that this self-assessment was key to fulfilling her true needs that weren't being met.

It may feel very uncomfortable to have to recognize, experience, or address certain feelings or situations. But until you do, you might keep using food to avoid them. So before you start eating, stop and ask yourself, "Why do I want to eat?" If you're not actually hungry, ask yourself, "What do I really need instead of food?"

Creating a list of what you CAN do to replace eating is KEY to changing your habits. We don't want to be left feeling bored, lonely, stressed, anxious, tired, or sad. If you just decide that you won't eat when you're not hungry, and you don't replace eating with a new habit, you'll still be stuck with those feelings and may eventually go back to comfortably using food to suppress those feelings. If you have intense feelings that cannot be appeased with a new habit, practice sitting with those feelings. It can be incredibly uncomfortable to experience sadness, frustration, loneliness, or pain but doing so allows you to be more aware of what you really need as opposed to using something to numb or distract from your true feelings. Acknowledging your feelings instead of suppressing them with food is the first step toward releasing them and creating change.

Sarah discovered that her poor eating habits were always in the evening. Sarah is a nurse and comes home to three needy children and a husband looking for her attention, too. After dealing with the pressure of her job, it's difficult to give her love and attention to the family. Sarah confessed that salty chips and a glass of wine (that turned into four glasses of wine) were her mental escape after a demanding day. I asked her to question what her mind and body are really telling her that she needs. I gave her the week to really think about it. When she came back a week later, she realized that she wasn't communicating her needs to her family. Instead, she was suppressing her feelings and using indulgences for pleasure. She had a talk with the family and they agreed to let her unwind with a 30-minute workout and a hot bath after. They also agreed to help get dinner started to take off some of the stress of evening duties. Understanding and communicating what she really needed entirely changed the outcome of her evening.

If you find that you are craving food when you're feeling stressed or sad, finding outlets of happiness or stress relief can be incredibly helpful and is the next step in freeing yourself of that emotion. Having a list of activities that you enjoy will help you break the habit of using food and enable you to create new habits instead. You will be finding new ways, other than food, to boost the neurotransmitters in your brain that make you happy. Serotonin is a neurotransmitter that researchers believe controls our mood. Many studies show a strong link between depression and low serotonin levels. When you eat carbohydrates, such as chips, cookies, desserts, and bread, insulin is secreted. Insulin allows the tissues in your body to use up both glucose and amino acids, except tryptophan. Tryptophan gets priority to go to your brain since it isn't busy being used up by other areas in your body. Tryptophan is then converted to serotonin and, just like that, the extra serotonin boosts your mood and gives you good feelings! Once your brain recognizes that carbohydrates amplify these good feelings, you begin to crave them more, perpetuating an addictive state. Drugs, such as ecstasy and LSD, also use a serotonin pathway to boost mood and create a euphoric experience.

As your body becomes used to this state, you increase your serotonin receptors, needing more of your "drug" the next time around. This explains why it is incredibly important to find healthy methods for boosting your serotonin to feel happy instead of using food. You will always want more. One study compared the addictive comparison between sweeteners and cocaine. Rats were offered sugar, the non-nutritive sweetener saccharin, and cocaine. Ninety-four percent of rats chose sugar and saccharin over cocaine. Another group of rats that were already exposed to cocaine with signs of addiction still chose the sugar or saccharin over cocaine. This can be a huge consideration for what processed sugar can do in our brain!

Exercise, outdoor activity, and exposure to sunlight have all been found to naturally increase serotonin levels. If you wake up without a little pep in your step, try to take a 20-minute walk for a serotonin boost to adjust your state of mind before the day begins. References for more information on serotonin and eating can be found at the back of the book.

As human beings, we are wired to desire love and affection. If we aren't getting it, we will find the next best thing to fulfill that need. Many people find that their loneliness, whether it be from a dull relationship or the lack of a relationship, is comforted by food. When a new relationship or love interest sparks again, all of the sudden they lose the desire and intimate relationship that they had with food. They are fulfilling that need in a whole new way. If your cravings are coming out of loneliness, I may not be a matchmaker or marriage counselor, but my suggestion to you is to find a positive way to bring love into your life. Food will never fully satisfy that need.

John was very enthusiastic about his health and was eating an impressively clean diet and exercising for about two hours every day. John only had one downfall. After his busy workday was done and get-togethers with friends were over, he went back home to be alone. He was eager to be married and have kids but it just hadn't happened for him yet. Just about every night he turned to ice cream and snacks to feel comforted. John realized that his sweet treats would never give him the love he was really looking for. He agreed to start doing evening yoga classes to meet new people and make more friends. And if that didn't work... well, John would be getting a puppy.

You might find love from a relationship, friendships, or even a new puppy, but fill your life with love and you won't need food to do it for you. Many have found that giving back to others was what they needed to find happiness and healing. Volunteering in community organizations in particular has been shown to create higher levels of life satisfaction, creating an effect on overall happiness and general physical well-being.

Allison was such a kind-hearted and hard-working woman. She worked long hours at an office Monday through Saturday while juggling graduate school at the same time. In my eyes, Allison really deserved Sunday off from work, but she confessed that she dreaded Sundays. She didn't have much to do on her only day off so she found pleasure in food to pass the time. I suggested a few things that she might like to do instead, like going for a walk or calling a friend, when a craving comes on. She agreed, but each week she admitted that she just couldn't do it. I felt a little stuck on how I could help her until one day she came into my office elated. I asked her how her weekend went and with a big smile, she said, "I did something different this time. There was a rally to support rights for gay, lesbian, bisexual, and transgender groups. It was such a fulfilling experience to be a part of something that is making a difference for other people." Allison learned that when she spent her free time giving back to others, she was so fulfilled that she didn't need food to do it for her.

Write a list of five things that make you happy which you could do instead of using food. These will be your "Food Fixes." It could be as simple as going for a walk, calling a friend, reading a book, taking a nap, exercising, a hobby you enjoy, or choosing from your list of what makes you happy in Part 2. When you see your trigger coming up, such as feeling bored, frustrated, or tired, you can prepare by using one of your five Food Fixes instead. Keep in mind that this task may be easier said than done and will most likely require plenty of practice.

My Food Fixes:

1. _____
2. _____
3. _____
4. _____
5. _____

Once you begin making your *Mastering Mindfulness Plan*, also consider the socially challenging situations that you listed in Part 2. If your inner circle of friends is constantly sabotaging your eating habits, I would recommend either letting them know your struggles and that you need their support or maybe find new friends. Try to encourage people around you to make adjustments that won't set you up to fail. Instead of meeting for drinks, try a new art class, workout class, or something else that doesn't put you in a vulnerable position. If you are going to a party and you know there will be a lot of indulgences, I highly recommend eating something first so you don't arrive ravenous. Hungry + a buffet + indulgent foods is a recipe for mindless disaster.

I used to always get nervous about the holidays because, by the time we got through appetizers, dinner, and long conversations with dessert on the table, we all left entirely stuffed and guilty. One year my family agreed to change up our typical tradition and start something new. We only made a few light appetizers instead of the massive spread we were used to and by the time dessert came around, we would have one serving then leave the table. Instead of sitting around mindlessly indulging, we would get up together as a family and go for a walk. We had little babies in strollers, moms, dads, aunts, uncles, cousins, grandma and grandpa, and even great-grandma, too. When the weather was particularly bad, we opted for a game of cards or charades. It became a much healthier tradition that created some of our best memories yet. Challenge your social norms and traditions to start creating an environment that will support your goals.

When you're ready to eat, practicing mindful eating will allow you to tune into your hunger signals to fuel your body with how much it needs, and to fully enjoy the experience of eating. Not counting calories or measuring portions may seem scary at first, but over time you'll learn to trust yourself again. Just like any bad relationship with poor communication, it takes time to rebuild trust. You may overeat when you first start practicing, but the more you practice, the easier it will get, until it becomes a natural habit.

Think of it as learning to speak a foreign language. In the beginning, it's going to be hard, as you have to think consciously about how to put the words together. But, with practice, it will slowly go from choppy and challenging to fluent and natural. It is all a learning experience, so don't give up if you find it difficult or that you're making mistakes.

Practicing mindful eating will allow you to feel full satisfaction from eating the foods you enjoy in moderate portions. Following these principles will allow you to eat according to your body's energy needs, without feeling deprived.

Practicing Mindful Eating

1. Before eating, take the opportunity to notice your hunger level and how you're feeling. Using the 1-10 rating scale can be helpful. Try to be in a calm and relaxed environment. Make the conscious choice to eat foods that are both nourishing and pleasing to you.

2. Make sure you're not distracted by the TV, phone, computer, etc. This is your meal time to really tune into your body.

3. Explore food using your senses: observe how it looks, tastes, and smells. Set a positive tone for the meal by having gratitude for the food that is about to nourish your body.

4. Take a bite and chew very slowly. For the first few times practicing this, close your eyes to really pay attention to the flavors. Put your fork down between bites and take your time. Sit back and relax and make sure your plate or bowl is resting on a table in front of you, instead of being held near your face.

5. About halfway through the meal, check in with yourself to assess your hunger level. If you feel full or satisfied, save the rest for later. You can always come back to it ANY time YOU feel hungry. No pressure to completely finish your plate. If you're still hungry, keep slowly eating and check in with your hunger levels along the way. Stop when you feel content.

If you're used to being a fast, distracted eater, mindful eating can be a challenge. Take the opportunity to practice during any meal or even snack time.

I recently spent time at a Buddhist monastery in Escondido,

California, to observe the real *masters of mindful eating*. We spent hours in the morning taking slow walks through the mountains and practicing meditation. My stomach burned and growled with hunger. I'm pretty sure at one point I imagined myself tackling one of those monks just to see if they were hiding a pocket full of tofu or something. I was near the point of "hangry zombie attack."

However, once I realized that I wasn't going to die of hunger, I stopped focusing on the anxiety of when I would get to eat. Instead, I practiced accepting this uncomfortable feeling, knowing that it is only temporary and I would be fed again soon. I learned to mentally slow down and take deep breaths to let go of the demands for immediately needing food when hunger comes on. When it was finally time for lunch, I was challenged to eat slowly, mindfully, and in control, knowing that I am not powerless over feelings of hunger. While my body wanted me to scarf down my food, I followed the monks, who chose to mindfully eat instead. Together, we ate slowly and savored the experience. Heightening my senses and practicing self-control brought an overwhelming feeling of gratitude for the food that was warm, flavorful, and nourishing in just the right amount. Not any more, not any less.

You may not go as far as eating like a monk, but a good way to start is by practicing mindful eating with one meal each day. If you are used to eating until your plate is empty, instead of listening to your hunger, challenge yourself to leave one bite of food on your plate. Emily Post, the goddess of manners, used to say it was good manners to leave just a bit on the plate. That showed you had been given more than a sufficient amount of food to be satisfied. Leaving a little bit of food is a reminder to start checking in with your hunger level, and the first step to being in control over your food instead of letting an empty plate tell you when to stop. The more you practice, the more you will have the control to stop at any point that you feel content.

Many people were raised with the idea that you need to

completely finish your plate. It's easy to have "eyes bigger than your stomach," so if you continue to use your empty plate as a cue for when to stop eating, you will almost always eat more than what your body actually needs. If you do finish your plate and you're still hungry, don't feel the need to challenge yourself to leave food. Go ahead and eat until you're truly satisfied. Feel free even to get seconds if your body is still signaling that you are hungry. As you keep practicing, you'll be able to eat until you feel just content, or slightly full. Mastering this technique plays a pivotal role in gaining control over your food.

If you're one of the many who eat in front of the TV, while working on the computer, while browsing through your phone, or with your head buried in a good book, I really urge you to practice dining without those distractions. It really isn't possible to fully enjoy the taste of your food and pay attention to your hunger and satiety signals if you're distracted. Have you ever watched a movie and before you knew it your hand was hitting the bottom of a snack bag? At some point, most of us have. Not only did you likely eat more than what your body needed, you also missed out on a lot of the enjoyment you get from savoring the flavor. It's like getting the calories but cheating yourself out of the wonderful experience of eating! Part of the reason why we are driven to eat is for pleasure. If you don't let yourself receive that pleasure from your meals, you are likely to wander back into the kitchen for more food until that need is met. It may feel less entertaining or productive to not have any distractions but commit to making it your meal time. Don't cheat yourself out of the satisfying experience that eating brings.

Eating slowly is key to giving your mind time to register that your stomach is full. It takes about 20 to 30 minutes for your stomach to send the signal that no more food is needed. If you quickly eat, polish off your plate, and then realize you are a extra full, slow down! That is a clear message that you are not giving your body enough time to send the signal to your brain that you have had enough food. If you're used to eating fast, changing this habit may be easier said than done. Some of my clients like to make this their only goal to focus on for a few weeks before moving on to any food-related changes. They find it is easier to slow down by practicing to set their fork down in between each bite or even eating with their other hand that they don't normally use. If you find your head hovering over your place with relentless fork-scooping, try setting down your fork in between bites, sitting back and relaxing, thoroughly chewing, and savoring each delicious bite.

There are no rules – you're 100 percent in control of when you choose to eat. Whether it's a few hours, one hour, or ten minutes after you last ate, you can eat anytime you feel hungry. That's your body's signal telling you it needs more fuel! Listen to it closely and you'll be able to manage your weight effortlessly. When you put diet rules and restrictions on your eating, you will feel the urge to clean your plate, not knowing when you'll be "allowed" to eat again. When you have the freedom to eat anytime you want, you're much more willing to set the food aside when you're content.

When you tell yourself, "I swear I will never eat another cookie or dessert again," all of a sudden that cookie becomes the focus. It always comes back to "you want what you can't have." When you set "can't have" rules, the level of desire goes up for a few reasons:

Directed attention: Once you "can't have it," the forbidden food is brought to your attention even more. From childhood to adulthood, we always want what we can't have.

Rules: No one actually likes to be controlled with rules. Give a teen a few rules and they will be quick to break them faster than when not having the rules. Most people would have heightened curiosity to peek behind a door if there is a sign reading "Do Not Open" versus a door with no sign.

Perceived scarcity: If you think you only have this one opportunity left to have a dessert, you're going to overindulge because you swear, "it's the last time ever." The study "War and Obesity: The Role of Eating Habits" found that those who were in regions experiencing World War II were linked to obesity in late adulthood. This is very likely because these regions endured food scarcity during the war, but after the war ended and these regions became more food-abundant, the feelings of scarcity remained.

Think about eating like a toddler. Before the environment influences a toddler, they are mindful masters! They don't care whether it is dinner-time or not; when they feel hungry, they want food! It also doesn't matter if they are eating the most amazing delicious pizza you could ever have. When they decide they are full, they stop eating. Tune into your inner child and practice listening to what it really needs. Disregard the time of day and try eating when your body sends you true hunger signals, and stopping when you feel content.

Mindful eating gives you the ability to indulge in desserts and treats without feeling that you need to overeat or binge; that's because you know you can have them at any time. You become empowered instead of feeling like a teenager with rules! Over time, you'll be in control over your food instead of your food controlling you. Food will become your fuel, not your enemy.

While mindful eating and rebuilding your relationship with food is the focus, healthy eating can help your body feel good and make *mastering mindfulness* MUCH easier. If you're eating foods that digest really quickly and are full of salt, sugar, and flavoring, it can be really difficult to eat slowly and in control. Highly palatable foods can even stimulate the hunger hormone ghrelin to override your satiety signals when you're full. This is why some people may not be triggered to overeat from stress, boredom, or other feelings, but still feel out of control. When eating your favorite indulgent foods, the appetite-stimulating hormone ghrelin can increase significantly and stay elevated for two hours after you start eating. So, eating highly processed, pleasurable foods could actually reprogram the way your brain/gut system works. Once you give in to the temptation, the addictive serotonin process of eating sweets and other refined carbohydrates also makes it feel impossible to stop. This is why practicing mindful eating is much easier when you are making healthier choices.

The following nutrition strategies can help you fuel your body while practicing mindfulness. As you begin to heighten your self-awareness, you can observe how your body responds to certain foods and eating patterns. There are many different approaches to healthy eating that all come with pros and cons. This is a basic guide for foundational healthy eating so keep in mind that you are unique and may need to customize these recommendations.

1. Strive for whole foods. Try to choose foods that are less processed with fewer additives. Get used to tasting the actual food instead of artificial flavorings that can send you out of control. You might be wondering, "What is considered a less processed, whole food?" A good guide is to first think about how many steps your food had to go through to get on your plate. For example, let's start with apple pie. By the time you add all the other ingredients and it goes through the baking process, there are not many nutrients left to count as your daily serving of fruit. The next better option would be applesauce. You might find two or three ingredients, hopefully coming from natural sources, but you lose a lot of the health benefits in the processing. The best option would be the whole apple. The whole apple is full of nutrients and antioxidants and doesn't have an ingredients list of additives and preservatives. It's only pure apple. Eating real whole foods can free your mind knowing that you are only consuming nourishing foods, so you can just enjoy the experience of eating.

2. Eat more food earlier in the day. Those who are struggling to eat mindfully often make the mistake of skipping meals, particularly breakfast. If you lose control and overeat later in the day, having a bigger breakfast or lunch or adding in more snacks throughout the day can make a big difference in normalizing your appetite later. Having no breakfast in the morning with uncontrollable cravings in the evening is a very common pattern for those struggling to eat healthfully at night. If you choose to skip breakfast, you aren't getting the fuel you need for the day. If you're not giving your muscles, organs, and brain adequate fuel you are likely going to feel sleepy, fatigued, foggy, and even cranky. It can also trigger those survival instincts to come out in the evening and create intense cravings, making you wonder why you can't stop. Eating breakfast gives your body the steady fuel it needs to stay energized and helps you feel satisfied throughout the day, which also helps you make sensible choices and eat mindfully in the evening. I consider a "big" breakfast to be about one-third of the amount of food I would eat in a day. There is no specific time that you have to start eating. Just know that you might need to eat more food earlier in the day if you feel out of control in the evening. If you don't feel hungry in the morning, it is most likely because you are still digesting food from the night before. Slowly practice adding a little bit of breakfast food at a time and gradually increasing the amount when you are able. For example:

Day 1-3: Whole grain toast
Day 4-5: Whole grain toast + avocado
Day 6: Whole grain toast + avocado + 2 hard-boiled eggs
Day 10: Whole grain toast + avocado + 2 hard-boiled eggs + 1 piece of fruit

By not skipping meals, many people find that uncontrollable evening snack habits naturally taper off making a substantial breakfast and lunch one of the key pieces in *mastering mindfulness.*

3. Choose healthy carbohydrates. Most find that the more refined sugar and sweets they eat, the more cravings they have. Carbohydrates provide a quick and easy source of fuel to our body in the form of glucose. When we eat highly refined carbohydrates and sugar, they digest quickly. That causes the sugar in our blood to spike, then drop relatively quickly. The bigger the fluctuations in blood sugar, the more likely you are to have carbohydrate cravings and lose control over food. This also puts the body under physical stress. Healthy sources of carbohydrates have more fiber than refined sources of carbohydrates. Fiber digests slowly, keeping you fuller longer and helping to prevent blood-sugar crashes. Whole grains, such as whole-wheat flour/bread/tortillas, quinoa, steel cut oats, and brown rice are good sources of fiber. Fiber is also found in the skin of fruits and vegetables and in nuts and seeds. Refined grains, such as white rice and bread, pasta, tortillas, English muffins, crackers, cookies, and bagels made of unbleached enriched flour, are stripped of their fiber. Therefore, simple carbohydrates and refined grains digest more quickly, often resulting in "crashing" and feeling hungry again not long after eating. Because whole grains digest more slowly, you will lessen the big insulin spike and the serotonin surge you get from refined carbohydrates. Another bonus: Fiber can lower cholesterol and keep the digestive tract healthy. Fiber adds "bulk" to the digestive system so if you are adding extra fiber to your diet, be sure to drink more water to keep the digestive system "moving." Remember, fiber is your friend.

4. Eat adequate protein. Protein also digests more slowly than carbohydrates alone. Most people find that when they switch from carbohydrate based snacks and meals to ones consisting of mainly proteins and fats, they feel much more satisfied and in control over the portion size. Instead of just having fruit, have fruit with a Greek yogurt, peanut butter, or a hard-boiled egg. Instead of having just popcorn, add in a few nuts and seeds for a slower digesting mix of carbs, fats, protein, and fiber. Adequate protein is also important because it is needed to maintain muscle mass. Muscle is a major source for the body to burn calories so having enough protein helps maintain a healthy metabolism. Try to make about one-fourth of your plate a protein source at each meal. Examples of healthy proteins could be quality lean meats, fish and seafood, lentils, beans, pumpkin seeds, hemp seeds, sunflower seeds, eggs, tempeh, tofu, and beans.

Charlene was a great example of how satisfying protein choices can be. She loved her morning ritual of two waffles with a little whipped cream on top. She couldn't figure out why she still felt ravenous all morning even though she already had breakfast. Charlene implemented these strategies by replacing one of the waffles for two eggs. She was able to still eat the waffle she loved and balance it with a protein choice. She found that adding the protein to her breakfast was key to feeling satisfied all morning, and it allowed her to have a sensible lunch.

If you're feeling ravenous after eating, make sure you've had a serving of protein. It might make all the difference!

5. Eat plenty of healthy fats. Eating fat does not necessarily create weight gain. Too much of any source of calories, whether it be from carbohydrates, protein, or fat, can cause weight gain. Fats are very satiating and are important for your brain health, nervous system, hormone production, absorption of some vitamins, and cardiovascular health. Fats that are less processed from whole foods offer the most health benefits, such as avocado, nuts, seeds, olives, olive oil, coconut oil, nut butters, and quality animal sources. Industrially produced fats that are designed to be shelf stable and highly palatable, such as trans-fats and hydrogenated oils, are detrimental to our health. These fats are found in some baked goods, fried foods, crackers, cookies, and other snack foods. Having healthy fats at each meal or snack can be a great way to feel more satisfied while keeping your body healthy.

6. Make half of your meal fruits and/or vegetables! Fruits and especially vegetables add bulk to your meals so you can have a much fuller plate for very few extra calories. A fuller plate will take longer to eat to give your gut/brain connection the time it needs to register that you are getting full. It is difficult to not over-consume calorie-dense foods if you're not having plenty of vegetables to bulk up the meal. Fruits and vegetables give you an array of nutrients that energize your body. The colors found in different fruits and vegetables provide a variety of health benefits so aim for five colors per meal.

A good goal is to strive to make half of your plate fruits and/or vegetables. If you're struggling to make half of your meal vegetables, start by looking down at your plate and asking, "What vegetables do I like that I could try adding to this meal? How many colors do I have on my plate and how could I add more variety that I like?"

Balancing your meals with one-fourth starch/grain, one-fourth protein, and one-half fruits or vegetables can take time and practice, so don't be too hard on yourself if your plate needs a little work!

7. Stay hydrated. Hunger and thirst signals both come from the hypothalamus in your brain, so you could be getting signals that you're hungry when you're actually thirsty. Dehydration can have significant effects on our health considering that about two-thirds of our body is made up of water. We need water for proper digestion and elimination, lubrication for the joints, good circulation, and the health of our skin and other organs. Dehydration can result in fatigue and sleepiness, headaches, muscle cramping, dizziness, decreased physical and mental performance and, in severe cases, unconsciousness. Ongoing dehydration can lead to kidney stones, constipation, and damage to the liver, joints, and muscles. A good rule of thumb is to strive to drink each day half of your body weight in ounces of water. It may sound like a lot of water to drink, but if you keep it handy throughout the day, you will be surprised at how easy it can be to reach your water goals. It can be helpful to listen to your body to see if you need more water, but try not to wait until you are already thirsty, as that is a sign that dehydration is already setting in. Sports drinks, fruit juice, soda, and some beverages other than water are often calorie-dense and contain added sugar or artificial sweeteners, flavorings, and/or colorings so it is not recommended to include them as your daily water intake.

For more nutrition strategies and recipes, go to www.Gina-B.com/members as a free resource to guide you.

Being prepared is also a big part of successfully *mastering mindfulness*. If you are going from meal to meal with little to no planning, you may end up too hungry without the right options ready. How can you practice mindfulness if you are in a hurry without anything planned and have to resort to quickly picking up a pizza instead? A common downfall comes from inadequate preparation and planning, causing impulse decisions. When most people hear the words "meal prepping," they picture thirty pieces of Tupperware and their entire Sunday spent in the kitchen, but it doesn't have to be that intense. Preparing could be as simple as going through your cupboards every Sunday to make sure you have all the food items on hand that you need for the week. If you don't have what you need, make a grocery list and hit the store. You could even get a little extra prepared by washing and chopping those fruits and veggies so they are ready to be cooked or snacked on throughout the week!

Susan had been diligently striving to prep and plan her meals. However, one day she worked much later than planned and drove home STARVING. Susan had definitely reached the level 1 "zombie attack" scenario and knew she was headed for trouble. When she got home, she ferociously opened the fridge and there it was... shining like a beautiful beacon of hope in all its glory: a bowl of pre-sliced watermelon. She had completely forgotten that she had planned ahead and had it chopped and ready. In that moment, it completely saved her from sabotaging her goals! She was able to mindfully enjoy a bowl of watermelon to hold her over while she cooked the healthy dinner she had planned. She also had a full container of vegetables washed and chopped, so it made cooking dinner a lot easier. If she didn't have the watermelon and veggies pre-washed and chopped, she probably would have gone back to her old ways and ravenously downed a bag of chips and lost her appetite for dinner.

You could take preparation one-step further by choosing which meal is most challenging for you to prepare and having a batch ready ahead of time. If you know that dinners are always your downfall because you're hungry, tired, and tight on time, you may want to prepare a batch of soup, stew, or something you can have throughout the week. I've actually had a client who knew that breakfast was his biggest challenge because his mornings started at 4:30 A.M. He easily fixed that problem by preparing thirty breakfast burritos and freezing them so he had a month's worth of breakfast ready to go! If you are ultra-ambitious, you could have breakfast, lunch, dinner, and snacks all prepared for the week. When you know that you have healthy options readily available, you will have much more confidence and trust that you will make better food choices. There is no right or wrong here. Just remember that failing to prepare is preparing to fail, so note what level works best for you. The more prepared you are, the more you can relax and mindfully enjoy a delicious and nutritionally balanced meal.

Now it's time to start creating your plan. Use the *Mindfulness Mastery Plan* in the back of the book to create your strategies for the mindful eating struggles that you have discovered. You may want to browse back through the Food Log in Part 2: Observing the Present to review your current eating habits and see what changes you want to be included in your plan. Looking back through Part 1: Exploring the Past may also help if you noticed that parts of your past influence your eating habits today. You may want to focus on letting go of ideas that you were raised with, such as finishing your plate, quickly eating, or feeling the need to sneak indulgences. If you have a comforting memory associated with a certain food, you may want to be very mindful when eating that food to make sure it isn't being used to cope. When creating your plan, make sure you write very specific solutions so you know exactly what actions to take. Here are examples of good and bad solutions:

Problem: Snacking in front of the TV.

A bad solution: Try not to overeat in front of the TV.

The above solution is too vague and doesn't give you a clear plan of action. Without clear direction, you are setting yourself up to fail.

A good solution: Eat a pre-portioned snack before sitting in front of the TV, or try a new evening activity instead to help disconnect the TV-snack habit.

Problem: I eat until I feel stuffed.

A bad solution: I won't eat so much.

A good solution: I will practice eating more slowly and setting my fork down in between bites to listen to my hunger at dinner each night this week.

See the difference? It is much easier to create a solution that is vague, but it's also the main reason why so many people never accomplish their goals. When they are faced with the moment of choosing their new solution or going back to their comfortable habit, the old habit will win because they don't know exactly what their plan of action is. The more specific your solution is, the easier it will be to choose the new habit instead of having to figure it out when you're vulnerable. The following charts are common problems and solutions that you can use to guide your thinking, but by no means are they complete lists.

Time

Problem: Large gaps in between meals causing overeating later.

Solutions:
- Have three to five meals per day so you don't go longer than four hours without eating.
- Bring portable snacks to eat as needed.

Problem: Focusing on time to eat instead of listening to hunger cues.

Solutions:
- Before eating ask, "Am I really hungry? Does my body need food at this time?"
- If not, find a distraction.

Food

Problem: Eating quantities that are larger than needed or undesirable food choices.

Solutions:
- Try eliminating specific trigger foods that are causing overeating until you regain trust and control.
- Be aware of the trigger foods for you; practice eating them mindfully.
- Try swapping foods you wanted to change for a healthier, less processed alternative.
- Make sure you are prepared with healthy options on hand.
- Have a mix of carbohydrates, fats, and proteins to feel more satisfied.

Hunger and Satiety

Problem: Starving before eating (hunger level = 1-2).

Solutions:

- Add a snack between meals so you don't get overly hungry and overeat at the next meal.
- Plan ahead with meals so you don't make impulsive food choices when hungry.

Problem: Feeling full or stuffed but overriding satiety and eating anyway (hunger level = 6-10).

Solutions:

- Before eating ask, "Am I really hungry?" Eating when not hungry indicates you want food for other reasons. Ask, "What do I really need?"
- Remove yourself from the area so you won't be tempted to mindlessly eat.

Problem: Feeling too full (hunger level 8-10) after eating.

Solutions:

- Practice eating slowly and putting your fork down in between bites.
- Challenging yourself to stop when you feel 80 percent full (hunger level = 6).

Activity

Problem: Engaging in activities that distract you while eating or from listening to hunger cues – TV, phone, computer, books, movies, driving, etc.

Solutions:

- Commit to turning off or removing distractions to give eating your full attention.
- Schedule lunchtime into your calendar so you don't have to work or multi-task during meals.

Problem: Overeating in social situations – group lunch, buffets, work gatherings, social events and holidays.

Solutions:

- Eat something before attending a social event so you aren't ravenous and tempted to overeat.
- Go for the fresh fruits and veggies and go lighter on calorie-dense appetizers and snacks.
- Make a plate... then step away from the buffet!
- Bring a healthy dish to pass so you're not held captive to party foods.
- Meet up with friends and do something not involving food.
- Remind yourself that just because a food is available to eat or for free, it doesn't mean you have to eat it if it sets you back from your goals.

Feeling

Problem: Feeling bored

Solutions:

- ➢ Download an audiobook and go for a walk.
- ➢ Find an enjoyable distraction or a new hobby.

Problem: Feeling tired

Solutions:

- ➢ Take a quick power-nap.
- ➢ Go for a walk to boost energy.

Problem: Feeling angry or sad

Solutions:

- ➢ Walk outside, play with pets, call a friend, breathe, observe emotions and watch them pass by, journal your feelings or situations, or find a healthy way to cope with emotions.

Problem: Feeling stressed

Solutions:

- ➢ Make a to-do list, brainstorm solutions to problems, meditate, exercise, take a bath, go for a walk, get a massage, do a quick stretch, unwind to music, laugh.

Your problems and solutions don't have to address all of these topics – just any that you feel are a problem for you. Again, make sure that your plan of action is very clear. Mindful eating solutions could pertain to meal prepping, listening to hunger cues, making healthier choices, trying other ways to cope with feelings, practicing mindful eating, etc. Create your Mindful Eating Plan now in the back of the book before moving on. Additional copies can be downloaded from www.Gina-B.com/book.

> "IT IS IN YOUR MOMENTS OF DECISION THAT YOUR DESTINY IS SHAPED."
> - TONY ROBBINS

Mindful Living

Now that you've observed what makes you feel stressed, you can practice making peace with or letting go of those situations that are out of your control and handle the rest with focus and clarity. Mental, emotional, or physical stress significantly increases the risk for developing numerous diseases. The effect of stress on eating habits varies from person to person. Some will overeat in response to stress and some lose their appetite. Regardless, the physiological impact of chronic stress is detrimental.

When you feel stressed, you're activating your *fight or flight* response. This releases cortisol, a hormone that increases blood sugar. This response was beneficial back in the caveman days when the blood sugar boost gave them extra energy to run from a wild animal. But if you are feeling stressed and not running from an animal (or finding a way to burn up the energy), the excess sugar will circulate throughout your bloodstream. If you are frequently putting your body in this elevated blood-sugar state, the sugar molecules are consistently rubbing against your arteries and increasing inflammation. This inflammation within the circulatory system increases the risk for diabetes and cardiovascular disease. Pair that chronic stress with a diet high in processed foods and a sedentary lifestyle and it could be deadly.

Staying in this *fight or flight* mode makes your adrenal glands work around the clock to create cortisol. If your cortisol is consistently high from stress or if you eventually overwork your adrenals until they are unable to make enough cortisol, you can end up with a hormone imbalance. Hormone imbalances are linked to insomnia, depression, low energy, an inability to focus, increased salt and sugar cravings, weight gain, a weakened immune system, and impaired digestion and/or digestive disorders.

Stress is also a significant focus for autoimmune disease

research. According to the peer-reviewed journal *Autoimmunity Reviews*, researchers suggest that psychological and physical stresses contribute to the development of autoimmune diseases. They predict that stress triggers the neuroendocrine hormones that regulate our immune system. This causes the immune system to go haywire and release cytokines, resulting in an autoimmune disease. Many studies have found that up to 80 percent of patients experienced uncommon emotional stress just prior to their disease onset. Over time, stress can take a significant toll on our eating habits, overall health, and happiness; so managing stress is imperative for prevention or treatment of any disease or illness.

A client of mine shared with me that her mother just turned ninety-seven without having any illness, isn't taking any medication, eats reasonably well but not super-healthfully, doesn't exercise at all, and yet is full of energy and still drives. I was shocked and had to know her secret. My client said, "She never takes anything too seriously. No matter what happens, she doesn't get stressed or hold onto it. I truly believe that is the key to life." After hearing her mother's story, I wasn't going to argue with that.

Some stress is out of our control, such as an ill family member, unexpected bills, and troubles at work or with the kids. Managing stress isn't about eliminating all stress but instead being aware of how you're letting your body respond to it. You may not be able to control the situation, but you can breathe through it to not let your body trigger the *fight or flight* response.

While our environment can't always be controlled, many of our worries and stresses are created by the little voice in our head that wants us to be entertained. Think of it as your own reality TV show. It might be garbage, but it's still entertaining! How many times have you worried about something that never happened? Have you ever sabotaged your goals and wondered if you do it because you would miss the rush of "starting over" again? Sometimes we create our own stress, anxiety, and self-sabotaging thoughts to fill the void or to make life a little more exciting. Recognize that you are not your mind. It is good to be aware of your thoughts and not use distractions to numb them, but know not to trust everything you think. Our mind is programmed to judge other people, overanalyze or misperceive situations, and worry about what has not yet happened. When you know that your mind sometimes creates irrational thoughts, you can resist its entertaining and ridiculous thoughts or attempts to sabotage your goals.

The Buddhists give great analogies as to how our mind is a garden. We are constantly planting new seeds. Your seeds might be worry, despair, suffering, anxiety, or loneliness. Or they might be peace, contentment, happiness, and positivity. Recognize what seeds you're planting in your mind and choosing to water and grow. When negative thoughts enter your mind, stop and ask yourself what you're cultivating within. Whether the stress in your life is within your control or not, how we handle it is most important.

Based on your journaling from Part 2: Observing the Present, what did you notice about how you handle situations or stress in your life? When you become more aware of your environment, you start to see how, and how often, you react. It's okay to respond, but an immediate reaction can trigger your cortisol stress hormones. Impulsive reactions never seem to help a situation, either. If you're driving and someone cuts you off, you may suddenly feel a surge of frustration. You might call them a jerk, or some other similar words, to yourself in the car. But has that ever changed the outcome of the situation? If it did, it probably wasn't for the better. The only thing that changed was your internal level of stress. When those feelings arise, try taking a five-second pause to refocus. Take a meditative moment to breathe and come back to reality. Take five deep breaths and ask yourself, "Does this stress really matter? Is this situation out of my control?" Take a moment to breathe through it and find your happy place again. Notice what seeds you are planting in your mind. It is easy to lash out and react if you are nurturing seeds of resentment, anger, or jealousy instead of compassion and understanding.

If you can influence the situation, take a few breaths and decide on the best option with clarity, not out of impulsive reaction. During this meditative moment, try heightening your senses. Can you feel your heartbeat, the wind in your hair, and the sun on your face? Can you smell flowers or food? Feel the tension starting from the top of your head, and visualize it melting away through your body. Focus on your breathing to help lower your heart rate so you don't spike your *fight or flight* hormones.

> *Liv4Yoga's meditation expert, Heather Foat, weighs in on how we can easily incorporate the principles of meditation into everyday life. Here are her insights on getting started:*
>
> *"Meditation doesn't need to be sitting on a cushion in some quiet space with no one around you. You can practice anywhere. Slow down and pause. Follow your breath. Pay attention to one inhale from beginning to end and an exhale from beginning to end. You did it! Now try that again and again when you walk, when you are sitting, or when you lay down, drive, talk, listen to someone, are in an argument, when you have a utensil in your hand. Pause and see for yourself what breath, mindfulness, and awakening to the moment can do for you. The key is to not overthink it and just breathe. Breathe long, full, deep, and conscious breaths to welcome yourself over and over again to the present moment."*

Can you calmly respond to situations without emotionally reacting? When people are rude, sarcastic, or hurtful, know that it is their personal problem and not yours to absorb and react to. At any moment, you have the choice whether or not to let others control your emotions. Choose happiness. Remember this affirmation, and when you are faced with a difficult situation, remind yourself, *I choose happiness*. When you look into the world, what situations can you observe without emotionally absorbing? Observation can give you the freedom to acknowledge and respond to situations without creating internal distress.

Meditation can be easier than you think and can be a powerful tool in staying calm, happy, and focused during your day. It could be as simple as taking a moment to refocus and set an intention. When you wake up in the morning, ask yourself, "What do I want to gain from my day?" That is what your intention is. Maybe you want to achieve a new accomplishment, appreciate a carefree moment, fix an old relationship or start a new one, feel energized, conquer a to-do list, be positive, do something for yourself, or do something for others. A new intention doesn't have to be created every day. Sometimes I stick with the same one to focus on for a few days, or I rotate between a few.

Directing your attention to what you want to gain from the day will guide you toward achieving it, especially when distractions throughout the day will attempt to pull you away from it. Remember the main rule when learning to ride a bike? Don't stare at what you don't want to hit! If you look at it, you will hit it. Just watch a kid learn to ride a bike, and you will see them slowly veer off and run into whatever they have their eyes set on. Setting an intention for your day will help you focus on what's important to you, and it will direct your thoughts and actions toward it throughout the day. In all avenues of life, failing to prepare is preparing to fail. When life tries to challenge you, you will be prepared with your intention to stay on course. Practice living with intention.

While you're setting your intention, remember what you are

grateful for. Having gratitude shifts your mind out of the dark and into the light. If you are feeling disappointed about your lack of making perfect food choices, be grateful that you have access to food and that you are taking the steps to move in the right direction. If you are feeling upset with someone in your life, remember the qualities that they have that you are grateful for. You will be much more likely to communicate with love and understanding, rather than anger and criticism. If you are unhappy with your physical appearance, be grateful that your body can move and is keeping you alive to experience the world. You will find yourself embracing all the wonderful things your body can do. Having gratitude shifts your mindset from the pessimistic point of view toward the optimistic that opens the door to any possibility. If you don't take the time to acknowledge what you do have and have accomplished so far, you will never be satisfied. You will never feel good enough and an underlying anxiety will remain. Gratitude takes your mind out of the dark and into the light.

At this time list ten things you are grateful for. It may take a few minutes to come up with ten of them, but writing them down can help you vividly see all that you are grateful for, instead of letting a few of them vaguely float around in your mind. You can always peek back at your list when you need it.

I am grateful for…

1. _____
2. _____
3. _____
4. _____
5. _____
6. _____
7. _____
8. _____
9. _____
10. _____

Remind yourself about what you are grateful for when you first wake up in the morning, throughout the day, and just before falling asleep. Keep gratitude at the forefront of your mind, and you will find yourself happier and more thankful for the little things that most people take for granted. Practice less complaining and more complimenting, less gossip and more love, being less hateful and more grateful. When you're faced with challenges during your transformation, remember what you are grateful for. Fill your heart with gratitude and watch your relationships, outlook on life, and abilities profoundly transform.

In Part 2, you came up with a list of what makes you happy. You can always change, add, or remove ideas from this list, but just make sure that you have one. Fitting in time for what makes you happy is incredibly important for managing stress and staying positive throughout life's challenges. You may notice that some days you feel more optimistic and other days may feel more challenging. Turn inward to try to understand what influences your happiness. Think about what habits you have on days that you are happy, and what happens on days that you feel are a struggle. Being aware of your daily habits is a significant piece to living mindfully. What daily habits make you feel successful? The definition of success should be based on your own perception. Success could pertain to physical, mental, emotional, or financial health or any areas in life that make you feel as though you are thriving. These could be the puzzle-piece habits that build your "bigger picture." Try to include all areas of your life in which you want to be successful. Below is an example:

I am successful when:

- I go to bed early and wake up early.
- I do some sort of daily activity or exercise.
- I stay set an intention and practice mindfulness.
- I plan and prepare my meals ahead of time and eat well.
- I save money to feel financially secure.
- I make my bed and keep my space organized and clean.
- I am doing good for others.
- I make a to-do list in the morning
- I read before bed

I have a whiteboard hanging in my bedroom, and on it I listed what makes me happy and successful. I see it first thing in the morning and last thing before bed as a reminder to keep doing what makes me a happier person. Doing this may seem trivial, but putting it right in front of my face guides my choices every day. When I don't feel like going to bed early, making my bed, or meal prepping, I remind myself that I'll be much happier in the near future if I do. The more I keep making those choices, the quicker I will build those habits that will shape my future. Whether you keep this list hanging on your wall or written in this book, keep it in the forefront of your mind as a reminder of what actions keep you happy and successful.

Make your list of daily habits that make you successful to direct your actions toward creating a life you want to have.

I am successful when…

1. _____
2. _____
3. _____
4. _____
5. _____
6. _____
7. _____
8. _____
9. _____
10. _____

For me, yoga has become a key component to managing stress and creating happiness within. When I was younger, I used to do yoga for a little exercise and to keep my flexibility. I thought that was the purpose of yoga. When I moved to San Diego, I really immersed myself into the yoga practice, which became a significant part of my journey toward mastering mindfulness. Yoga didn't just bring me exercise; it brought me peace. It gave me sixty minutes to tune into my mind and body to explore what I really needed in that moment, without a cell phone or distractions. I could actually feel where my body was holding onto tension and let it release. Some days I learned that I needed movement to bring me energy, and other days I just needed stillness to breathe through stress. When life felt chaotic, my mat gave me comfort and safety. If my mind started to wander to people or situations that I was dealing with, the four corners of my mat blocked them out and didn't let them in. It was my personal time and space to reconnect with myself and free my mind of the influence that others imposed on my emotions. At the end of my session, I would leave re-centered and filled with positivity and happiness. I now consider yoga to be a date with myself.

For you, it might not be yoga, but set aside the time to listen to your needs without distractions or multi-tasking. Creating space to be alone is a key component to managing stress and creating happiness within. If you're constantly running errands, working, and entertaining your brain, you might forget to take the space to listen to your needs and understand yourself better. Make it a priority to give yourself at least ten minutes of quiet time to listen to what you need. You might learn where your body is holding onto tension or stress, and if you really need movement or stillness or to explore any thoughts you haven't had time for. Remember that health is the relationship between your mind and body. Take the personal time and space to reconnect with yourself and free your mind of the influence that others imposed on your emotions. Consider it a date with yourself to get to know you better.

Try to set aside the time to listen to your needs without music, a phone, people, or other distractions. It could be a brief meditation, a walk outside, a warm bath, or wherever you find silence to check in with yourself to see what you need. It is truly in moments of silence and solitude that we can hear our inner voice loud and clear, speaking for what it needs. If you have kids, it's okay to schedule a few minutes, or sixty, that are just for you. Even if you only have two minutes of free time, take a peek in the mirror and say, "Hey, how are YOU doing today?" Learn what will truly serve you in that moment. You might need movement and activity or you might really just need sleep.

When it comes to exercise and activity, having a structured plan can help you stick to your goals, but it's also important to ebb and flow with what your mind and body are telling you they need. I call it *Mindful Exercise*. You might originally plan to do a cardio workout one day, but when the time comes you might need to feel energized and powerful from strength training instead. Or you might plan to strength train but find that you need to work out a little stress with an intense cardio session. Or you might plan to do a slow yoga stretch but want to do a fun dance class instead. If you listen to what your body really needs and keeps you energized, you won't want to quit. If you feel like you're suffering on the treadmill every day and absolutely hate it, it's probably not going to be the tool that will keep you healthy for the rest of your life.

Think of it similar to the way you eat and ask, "Would I want to keep exercising this way forever?" Now, if your mind is telling you, "I need couch time and pizza!" every day, you may need a little more discipline and structure. Challenge yourself, but also tune into what you need so you stay energized, positive, and fulfilled. Keep in mind that regularly exercising or doing something active can help you become more in tune with your body and what it really needs. If you're not very active to begin with, starting an exercise program can feel challenging. But, just like practicing to incorporate better eating habits, it will eventually feel more natural and enjoyable.

It's easy to get so caught up and busy with life that we forget to take the time to disconnect from the outside world and live in the present moment. When we are patiently waiting at a stoplight, doctor's office, or having a meal alone, most people are quick to pull out their phone for mind-numbing entertainment. We're addicted to our electronics to distract us from reality and the experience of our own company that we find so unamusing. Even when we do have others around us, many will give in to the temptation of multi-tasking with social media and texting. We've become so consumed with the electronic world that we have to create new technology just to detox from our technology.

> *Zack Prager, expert in positive psychology and founder of the "disconnect to connect" mobile app Ransomly, gives his perspectives:*
>
> *"There are a lot of benefits of our hyper-connected lives. We have all the world's information in the palm of our hand. We can order pizza from bed with a click, we can share our lives instantly, and the list goes on. That hyper-connectivity comes at a cost, though. We often find ourselves more disconnected from each other. If you don't regularly and intentionally set aside a time and place to unplug, you are going to miss out on a lot of real moments in your life."*

You can't *master mindfulness* if you always fill the quiet moments with distractions. Challenge yourself to enjoy your own company, check in with your needs, and quietly observe what is going on around you. If you start to feel your mind racing with the day's to-do list, draw your awareness back into the present moment. Don't cheat yourself from enjoying your present by worrying about a future that doesn't exist yet. When you are more aware you can enjoy exploring your mind, appreciating the little things around you, or the company of the people you are with. When you are with your friends, family, or even talking with strangers, show them your gratitude and give them your undivided attention. Listen to them speak as though no one else in the world existed. Being present creates deeper relationships and gratitude for the moment.

Many people find that being out in nature fulfills their needs by putting their problems in perspective. Seeing the stars in the universe, a vast ocean or body of water, mountains on the horizon, a towering forest, or any space to immerse yourself in nature's beauty can make you feel so small. Having this new perspective may help you realize that maybe some of your problems aren't as grand as you originally supposed. The very stars that you are seeing may not even exist anymore by the time the light reaches your eye. The people who are long gone, but who were once standing on the same land that you are on now, also had their own problems and stress. One day, we will all be gone too. So, really evaluate… does this stress really matter? Do you make time to disconnect, be present, and do what brings you happiness? Always go back to your list.

Remember to set an intention for your day. Practice letting go of situations or emotions that do not positively contribute toward that intention. Do things to help you listen to your needs and bring you happiness. You may be holding onto resentment or anger from a past situation that happened or an apology you never received. Practicing forgiveness doesn't give permission for others to have done what they did, but it frees us from carrying the emotional burden they created. Get it out of your body and let it go. Try to make peace with, or address, difficult situations so you don't internalize them, suppress them, or use food or other pleasures to numb them.

Use the Mindfulness Mastery Plan at the end of the book to create personalized solutions for the mindful living struggles that you have discovered. You might find it useful to use some of the habits that make you successful as solutions. Here are some common problems and solutions that may also be helpful:

Mindful Living

Problem: Feeling a lack of purpose or motivation from your day.

Solutions:

- Start each morning by setting an intention for what you wish to gain or accomplish from the day.
- Start a goal book,

Problem: Feeling stressed with work, to-dos, etc.

Solutions:

- Take a few breaths or a moment for meditation.
- Set or return to your intention for the day.
- Make a detailed to-do list.
- Ask, "Is this situation within my control? Do I need to address it or let it go? Am I reacting or responding?"
- Schedule time in your calendar for your "happiness habits."
- Communicate your needs with others and ask for help when needed.

"I LET GO OF WHAT
NO LONGER SERVES ME,
TO MAKE ROOM FOR WHAT INSPIRES ME."

Mindful Self-Talk

Now that you've observed how you talk to yourself, how can you change your thoughts to help you become your best self? Most people think they need to talk down to themselves in order to stay disciplined and, if they have positive, self-loving thoughts, then they won't try hard enough to make changes. This is simply not true. If a young child is struggling in school and you constantly call them a failure, will that help them succeed? Probably not. With encouragement and praise for their small accomplishments, they'll begin to excel. Negative affirmations will create negative outcomes, whereas positive affirmations will create positive outcomes.

Still don't believe me? Consider this: What if you went into a coma and came out with no memory of your past. Your family tells you that you have been a sidewalk sweeper for the majority of your life, and you're back to work tomorrow! Would you feel very driven and motivated to succeed in your job? Now, what if they told you that you're a high-ranking political leader or the Queen of England, and the world needs your knowledge and skills to make important decisions. How do you think those two different scenarios would influence your motivation and self-confidence to create change and make accomplishments?

Change begins with our state of mind, and our state of mind is created by how we talk to ourselves. Naturally, our mind wants to direct our actions toward what is safe and comfortable, also known as the path of least resistance. In order to re-direct our actions, we truly have to believe that we are already who we are striving to be and our actions will follow. Otherwise, our mindset will continuously sabotage our goals as a protective mechanism from uncomfortable change. We *must* have a mental shift in order to have a profound change.

Look over what you observed about your self-talk from Part 2.

What if you said those same things to someone you really loved, like a close family member or your best friend? How would it make them feel? Do you think it could create a personal setback and lack of confidence? This should make you realize how incredibly important it is to be aware of your self-talk and how it influences your abilities.

Be aware that your environment can also have a huge influence on how you create your self-talk. It can be difficult to feel full of self-love when images of perfectly sculpted bodies are filling up Facebook, Instagram, and magazines. Fitter and healthier media celebrities can offer a lot of motivation, but they can also do a lot of harm if they create comparisons. If you are constantly comparing yourself to images of perfection, you will only be left feeling "flawed." It is easy to think that images of health gurus create positive inspiration, but often they create bitterness when we use them as a means of comparison. Self-shaming thoughts will never give the true motivation for change and will only feed the Destructive Self-Sabotaging Cycle. Instead of focusing on the gap between someone else's perfect body and your own, shift your mindset inward to the progress your own body is making. You will find yourself letting go of bitterness and filling yourself with gratitude to keep your momentum moving forward.

When I was going through my difficult life transition, my mind was filled with self-doubt and shame for my failures. I knew I needed to heal the relationship within myself before I could create the positive, thriving life that I wanted to have. I decided to write myself a love letter to finally make peace with the inner battle. I never in my life planned to share it with a single soul, but I feel deeply connected to each person reading this book and hope you feel inspired by my healing process.

Dear Gina,

I know it's been a while since we have talked, so I am trying to get reconnected. You have been through so much lately and have felt lost along the way, but I am proud of you for being brave.

You have had the courage to let go of toxic people you were addicted to and gave yourself the freedom to find you. I know you're scared but let go and be free. If you make the wrong decision, we will get through it together.

I'm sorry for all the bad things I've said about you. You never deserved it and I promise to only say all the amazing things you deserve to hear. I promise to love and cherish you and treat you as the goddess you are. I promise to fuel you and keep you active, inspired, and striving for your best to feel your best. I will respect you and let go of judging you. You are unique and amazing.

It's been a long road together, but I am learning how to trust you and listen to you better. Thank you for setting aside the time to get to know me better and not look at your phone while texts buzz off. I know some days we feel like soul mates and other days like strangers, but I'm here to discover you non-judgmentally. Because deep down, there's no one who gets me like you do. You are my only one.

Love,

    Gina

When I wrote this letter, I had no idea that it would have such a profound impact on my life. I frequently reflect on the words that I wrote to myself and try my best to keep my promises. In the past, you may have made mistakes or didn't treat your body with the utmost respect and love, but at some point, you have to forgive yourself and move forward. Putting my internal turmoil on paper allowed me to finally release the negativity and love myself again. This letter was truly the foundation for me to become highly self-aware during my own journey in *mastering mindfulness*. If past mistakes or struggles have left you with self-doubt and shame, it's time to heal the relationship within to believe that you can change your future. If you feel compelled to do the same, please feel free to use the next space:

Letter to Myself...

If being kind and encouraging to yourself is difficult at first, give it away to others. When we give love, we get love in return. Start by complimenting friends, family members, or even strangers. Maybe they look particularly well-dressed one day or you want to give encouragement to someone who is making a healthy choice by taking the stairs. Helping others have more confidence will help you start to build your own. When you give love and support to others, you will find it comes back around to you tenfold. When you do receive a positive compliment, try to genuinely accept it. Let the positivity become who you are. When we brush it off or say, "Thanks, but...," it's like giving back a gift. It pulls your mindset back to your "old self" and old ways.

When you are ready to change your self-talk, you can start by practicing "thought-stopping." When negative thoughts come into your head, just STOP! Say, "No, I will not think those thoughts that will only set me back." The first step is being aware of those thoughts and knowing that they are only destructive. As you become more mindful of your self-talk, you'll become a pro at thought-stopping. Once you are comfortable with blocking out hurtful statements, try replacing them with positive statements instead. The more you fill your mind with positive affirmations about who you are, the closer you will be to becoming the transformed person you are striving to be.

Visualize what you want every single day and believe that you are already there. When you create the vision in your mind of the person you want to be, your thoughts will lead you toward it. Your actions are merely the expression of your thoughts and beliefs so choose your thoughts wisely. In order to change, you have to deeply believe in your heart that you are worthy of the better life you want. You have to make the conscious decision and commitment that you are not the person of your past; you are the person that you choose to create.

Use the *Mindfulness Mastery Plan* in the back of the book to create personalized solutions for the *mindful self-talk* struggles that you have discovered. Here are some common problems and solutions that may be helpful:

Mindful Self-Talk

Problem: Feeling guilty after eating too much food, or indulgent foods.

Solutions:

- Remind yourself that indulgences can be a part of a healthy and balanced diet.
- Use it as a learning experience.

Problem: Having negative thoughts about the way you look.

Solutions:

- Practice thought-stopping by saying, "No! I will not talk to myself that way."
- Say positive, self-loving affirmations, such as, "I am thankful for my body that allows me to move and do the things I love to do."
- Remember that it is a journey and remind yourself that even if you have not completely accomplished your goals, every day you are making progress.

Practice, Learn, Grow

During every second throughout life you are evolving. Keep tuning inward to listen better and understand deeper. Don't ever give up on building the intimate relationship with yourself because, at the end of the day, you are all that you have.

Continuously work toward these life changes and never forget to celebrate the tiniest of achievements. Each time you build on a new accomplishment, you are adding another piece to create life's beautiful puzzle. The more you celebrate the "wins," the more motivated you will become to continue to create them.

While the information in this book is valuable, it isn't enough to create change if you don't implement what you've learned. Take time every day to practice your plan without judgment. *Mastering mindfulness* is not a destination to reach, but a journey to be enjoyed.

"WHEN LIFE IS SWEET, SAY THANK YOU AND CELEBRATE.

WHEN LIFE IS BITTER, SAY THANK YOU AND GROW."

– SHAUNA NIEQUIST

Even though you have finished this book, I am here for you every step forward. There are a few ways you can continue your journey:

1. Request to join our private Facebook support group. *Mastering mindfulness* isn't easy so don't go at it alone! Get additional support with new strategies and extra accountability from a community of people on the same journey as you. To request access, go to:

www.Facebook.com/groups/MasteringMindfulnessGroup

2. Dig deeper into nutrition strategies by joining the free membership at www.Gina-B.com/members. It is full of cutting edge nutrition research, recipes, and meal-planning ideas.

3. Download additional copies of the food log, journal sections, or Mastering Mindfulness Plan to continue your self discovery and make progress on your goals.

4. Book Gina B for an in-person *Mastering Mindfulness* program or speaking session for the real interactive and life-changing experience! Contact: Info@gina-B.com

FAQ

If I want to follow a structured meal plan or diet, can I still master mindfulness?

Yes! I don't recommend very low-calorie diets because eventually your inner instincts come out and make it very difficult to eat mindfully. However, if you choose to follow a meal plan for weight loss or specific dietary needs, practicing mindfulness is still very important to keep a healthy relationship with your body and needs.

Once I make my Mindfulness Mastery Plan, how long will it take?

It really depends on each person and where they are starting. Some people diligently practice and make significant progress in the first two weeks. Some may need a few months or years. I know that may sound like a long time, but if you have spent your entire life instilling bad habits, it could take some time to create and sustain new ones. Be patient, and remember it is a progressive journey. However, the more you practice, the quicker you will see changes.

I don't trust myself without calorie counting or rules. Will I overeat by giving myself permission to eat?

You might at first, but don't let it deter you from giving up food rules. Be easy on yourself if you overeat at first, and use it as a valuable learning experience. The more in tune you become with your body, the easier it will get not to overeat.

I messed up and overate! Should I eat less tomorrow to make up for it?

Try to go back to your normal way of eating by listening to your hunger cues. The most important thing is to keep working on the relationship and connection between your mind and body. You don't want to get pulled back into the big rollercoaster effect from overeating and restricting. Don't punish yourself with restriction. Be kind and remember that overeating can be a valuable learning experience to help you better understand your struggles and prepare you for the future.

I did the journaling, I practice, and I STILL feel out of control! What do I do now?

If you continue to practice and you still can't gain control you're your eating habits, don't be afraid to seek additional help from a therapist or health professional. Conquering your inner battles may not be as easy as resolving them in a journal. Some medical conditions, such as hormonal imbalances and blood sugar issues, can contribute to uncontrollable cravings and may therefore need additional help from a qualified health professional.

Mindfulness Mastery Plan

Key points to remember:

- *When creating your plan, be very specific with your problems and solutions.*
- *Let go of having the "perfect diet" mentality.*
- *Practice mindful eating.*
- *Use effective strategies or activities that make you happy in situations where, in the past, you've used food to cope.*
- *Set an intention for the day.*
- *Take small meditations.*
- *Practice thought-stopping and use positive affirmations.*

Mindful Eating

Problem	Solution

Mindful Eating

Problem	Solution

Mindful Living

Problem	Solution

MINDFUL LIVING

Problem	Solution

Mindful Self-Talk

Problem	Solution

Mindful Self-Talk

Problem	Solution

Bibliography

Danese, A., & McEwen, B. S. (2012). Adverse childhood experiences, allostasis, allostatic load, and age-related disease. *Physiology & behavior*, *106*(1), 29-39.

Fletcher B, Pine KJ, Woodbridge Z., & Nash A. (2007) How visual images of chocolate affect the craving and guilt of female dieters. *Appetite*, 48(2), 211-217. doi:10.1016/j.appet.2006.09.002

History of Mindfulness: From East to West and From Religion to Science. (2017, March 14). Retrieved June 13, 2017, from https://positivepsychologyprogram.com/history-of-mindfulness/

Klein, K., & Bratton, K. (2007). The costs of suppressing stressful memories. *Cognition & Emotion,21*(7), 1496-1512. doi:10.1080/02699930601109523

Kringelbach, M. L., & Berridge, K. C. (2010). The Neuroscience of Happiness and Pleasure. *Social Research*, *77*(2), 659–678.

Lengacher, C. A., Kip, K. E., Post-White, J., Fitzgerald, S., Newton, C., Barta, M., . . . Klein, T. W. (2011). Lymphocyte Recovery After Breast Cancer Treatment and Mindfulness-Based Stress Reduction (MBSR) Therapy. Biological Research For Nursing, 15(1), 37-47. doi:10.1177/1099800411419245

Lenoir M, Serre F, Cantin L, Ahmed SH. Intense Sweetness Surpasses Cocaine Reward. Baune B, ed. *PLoS ONE*. 2007;2(8):e698. doi:10.1371/journal.pone.0000698.

Ma, S. H., & Teasdale, J. D. (2004). Mindfulness-Based Cognitive Therapy for Depression: Replication and Exploration of Differential Relapse Prevention Effects. *Journal of Consulting and Clinical Psychology,72*(1), 31-40. doi:10.1037/0022-006x.72.1.31

Momeni, J., Omidi, A., Raygan, F., & Akbari, H. (2016). The effects of mindfulness-based stress reduction on cardiac patients blood pressure, perceived stress, and anger: a single-blind randomized controlled trial. Journal of the American Society of Hypertension,10(10), 763-771. doi:10.1016/j.jash.2016.07.007

Monshat, K., Khong, B., Hassed, C., Vella-Brodrick, D., Norrish, J., Burns, J., & Herrman, H. (2013). "A Conscious Control Over Life and My Emotions:" Mindfulness Practice and Healthy Young People. A Qualitative Study. Journal of Adolescent Health, 52(5), 572-577. doi:10.1016/j.jadohealth.2012.09.008

Mrazek, M. D., Franklin, M. S., Phillips, D. T., Baird, B., & Schooler, J. W. (2013). Mindfulness Training Improves Working Memory Capacity and GRE Performance While Reducing Mind Wandering. Psychological Science, 24(5), 776-781. doi:10.1177/0956797612459659

Owens, M. J., & Nemeroff, C. B. (1994). Role of serotonin in the pathophysiology of depression [Abstract]. Clinical chemistry, 40(2), 288-295. Retrieved June 13, 2017, from http://clinchem.aaccjnls.org/content/40/2/288/tab-article-info

Stress effects on the body. (n.d.). Retrieved June 13, 2017, from http://www.apa.org/helpcenter/stress-body.aspx

Stojanovich, L. (2010). Stress and autoimmunity [Abstract]. *Stress and autoimmunity, 9*(5), a, 271-276. doi:10.1016/j.autrev.2009.11.014

Veer, E. V., Herpen, E. V., & Trijp, H. C. (2015). Body and Mind: Mindfulness Helps Consumers to Compensate for Prior Food Intake by Enhancing the Responsiveness to Physiological Cues. *Journal of Consumer Research, 42*(5), 783-803. doi:10.1093/jcr/ucv058

Vengel, D. (2016). The relationships among mindfulness, rumination, and stress-related sleep disturbance (Doctoral dissertation, Alliant International University).

Wurtman, R. D., & Wurtman, J. J. (1986). Carbohydrate Craving, Obesity, and Brain Serotonin [Abstract]. Appetite, 7, 99-103. Retrieved June 13, 2017, from https://www.ncbi.nlm.nih.gov/pubmed/3527063.

Young, S. N. (2007). How to increase serotonin in the human brain without drugs. *Journal of Psychiatry & Neuroscience : JPN, 32*(6), 394–399.

Young, S. N. (1993). The use of diet and dietary components in the study of factors controlling affect in humans: a review. *Journal of Psychiatry and Neuroscience, 18*(5), 235–244.

Made in the USA
San Bernardino, CA
21 February 2018